RAMSAY'S DISEASE

Myalgic Encephalomyelitis (ME)
And the Unfortunate Creation of 'CFS'

Lesley O. Simpson Ph.D.
With
Nancy Blake B.A. C.Q.S.W.
UKCP-Accredited Psychotherapist

Experience, Comments, Controversies
Including
Suggestions for Managing Your Own Progress

LIFELIGHT
PUBLISHING

Published by Lifelight Publishing 2013
www.lifelightpublishing.com

Designed by Grainger Graphics

Copyright © Nancy Blake 2013
www.nancyblakealternatives.com

British Library Cataloguing in Publication Data. A catalogue record for this book is available from the British Library.

ISBN: 0-9571817-2-8
ISBN-13: 978-0-9571817-2-4

10 9 8 7 6 5 4 3 2 1

DEDICATIONS

From Les:

To Dr. A. Melvin Ramsay.
"...The failure to agree on firm diagnostic criteria has distorted the data base for epidemiological and other research, thus denying recognition of the unique epidemiological pattern of myalgic encephalomyelitis." - Dr. A. Melvin Ramsay

From Nancy:

To those without whom this book would not have seen the light of day: Sue Walsh, Tony Blake, and Phil Grainger.
And all of those whose kindness, generosity and physical help over the years has allowed me to become well enough to put it together. You know who you are.

CONTENTS

RAMSAY'S DISEASE

Myalgic Encephalomyelitis (ME)

And the Unfortunate Creation of 'CFS'

The main objectives of this book are threefold. Firstly, to eliminate the nomenclatural problems which have been a source of confusion for ME, by making it plain that Ramsay's Disease does not equate with terms such as ME/CFS, CFS/ME or ME/CFIDS. Secondly to recognise the contribution to research which Dr. A. Melvin Ramsay made in the general field of ME. From the viewpoint of an ME sufferer, it is rather tragic that his concepts of ME are virtually disregarded by modern workers. Thirdly, to provide ME people with information to help them understand the nature of their problem and to identify the lifestyle changes needed to improve their quality of life. (Note that at this time it is inadvisable to use the term "cure.") I apologise for the fact that for many ME people the more technical parts of the text may be heavy going, but I urge them to try to cover these parts at their own pace.

The book also includes, as a separate but integral component text contributed by Nancy Blake, a practising psychotherapist whose personal encounter with ME as a sufferer has given her both direct insight and a deep interest in the subject. As a psychotherapist, she knows that ME is not a psychological problem. She tells her own story, explaining how the information elsewhere in the book relates to her experience of the illness, in the hope this may make the technical aspects easier for other ME people to understand and take in. Nancy's contribution is distinguished by sans-serif text, and is included within boxes within my chapters.

My bibliographic references, denoted by numbers in (round brackets), are collected at the end of each of my chapters. Nancy's references are collated at the end of the book, and denoted by [square brackets].

Dr. L. O. Simpson

AN EXPLANATION OF THE BOOK

Nancy: The title of this book, 'Ramsay's Disease (ME)', is the name Dr. Simpson would like to see used to replace the ever more confusing titles given to this illness: Chronic Fatigue Syndrome and its variants being the most common. These titles are misleading because they include a wide range of other conditions under the various headings, invalidating both research results and treatment recommendations.

Why 'Ramsay's Disease?' In 1955, around two hundred and ninety staff members of the Royal Free Hospital in London all succumbed to an illness which had hitherto been relatively unknown, although other epidemics and individual cases were subsequently identified.

A virologist at the Royal Free, Dr. Malcolm Ramsay, became extremely interested in trying to understand the illness. He spent the rest of his career studying it, and trying to learn in detail about the nature of this extremely debilitating condition. He set out clear diagnostic criteria, and believed the illness to be what had previously been called 'benign myalgic encephalomyelitis' (The term 'benign', for an illness that is hardly benign, had arisen during the polio era, to distinguish it from poliomyelitis, because unlike the latter, it did not result in permanent paralysis. This word has subsequently been dropped). As a mark of respect for Dr. Ramsay's work, Dr. Simpson proposes reverting to Ramsay's original diagnostic criteria [1], and giving myalgic encephalomyelitis the name 'Ramsay's Disease'.

In the course of Dr. Ramsay's investigations, he identified about ninety of the original cases as atypical, possibly having a psychiatric component, and he eliminated them from his future studies.

To his lasting regret, he agreed to the request of two psychiatrists, Beard and McEvedy to be allowed to conduct research into the epidemic. [2] After consulting the notes of a selected group of patients, which included those Ramsay had eliminated, they published a paper proposing that the entire epidemic was a case of mass hysteria [3]. In support of this hypothesis they noted that most of the sufferers were female, and that previous outbreaks of hysteria had been recorded in enclosed communities of young and poorly educated women. Despite the fact that, along with other weaknesses in their article, nurses and doctors employed in a busy hospital in London do not seem to fit this categorisation very closely, their hypothesis was immediately accepted as being valid by the medical establishment, the media and the general public. In the forthcoming decades, the belief that ME was a simply a matter of hysteria defined both popular and medical attitudes toward people with ME.

Despite literally thousands of research papers showing physiological abnormalities in people who have ME, this psychiatric perspective – that ME is a product of 'faulty beliefs' – is still influential today. It is promulgated mainly by Professor Simon Wessely and his colleagues (who have been called 'the Wessely group'), and it is reflected in the fact that the 'specialist centres' set up by the NHS to help people who have ME are largely staffed by psychiatrists, psychologists, occupational therapists, and even people who specialise in sports psychology [4]

As a person who is almost recovered from ME, I have followed the history of this illness and its treatment in the U.K. for a number of years. This includes my practice of writing letters to various news media and journals in an effort to counter the opinions promulgated about ME by this powerful psychiatric lobby.

Dr. Simpson saw one of my letters and responded by writing directly to me, telling me about his extensive research with blood samples from people with ME, and we began a correspondence. When he told me that he had written a book about ME which had not been published, I naively assumed that uploading a book onto a self-publishing site would be a simple task, and I offered to do this. He then suggested that I contribute the story of my experiences with ME, and some of my thoughts about it, and incorporate those into the book as a co-author. As a result, the book consists of a mixture of the text of his original manuscript and my contributions and comments. This has all proved, predictably, to be much more complicated than either of us envisaged!

You are interested in this book because you want to learn more about ME, perhaps because you have ME, or are helping someone who does, or maybe you are in a profession which involves working with ME. Having explained how the book came about, I hope it will be helpful to you if I provide an explanation of its structure, and give some directions about where to go to find the particular information you are most interested in. I have attempted to make the readers' task easier by using different type styles to distinguish between Dr Simpson's material and mine, so that you will be able to identify each of our 'voices' throughout the text.

Where to begin? Let's start at the most basic level. Physiologically, one of the most fundamental processes necessary to our physical survival, and to the functioning of every, cell, tissue and organ in our bodies, is the delivery of oxygen and the removal of waste products. This work is performed by our red blood cells. The behaviour of blood as a fluid suspension — haemorheology – has been the subject of Dr. Simpson's research over many years, and in particular, he has investigated how variations in the shapes of red blood cells can influence their ability to traverse the body's capillaries in order to perform their vital functions. Clearly, this is a matter of immense importance for normal health. Yet the study of haemorheology has no place in medical textbooks or medical training.

Medical dogma holds that all red blood cells are biconcave discocytes – flat round shapes with an indentation in each side. Biconcave discocytes are highly deformable, enabling them to curl up and traverse tiny capillaries one-third their diameter. Dr. Simpson's researches (over 120 papers and one book) have demonstrated, however, that in many chronic conditions, the red blood cell population contains a high percentage of irregularly shaped red blood cells, which are stiff (non-deformable) and therefore unable to traverse the capillaries, depriving various tissues and organs of oxygen, and allowing waste products to accumulate. Thus, in any medical condition in which the shape population of red blood cells becomes dominated by irregularly-shaped ones, there will be symptoms caused by oxygen-deprivation and failure of the removal of waste products from areas of the body which are served by the capillaries. As Dr. Simpson has shown, one such condition is ME.

My strong conviction, supported by some observations in research papers [5], for example, is that, due to the effects of the shape changes in the red blood cell population, ME is characterised by the failure of the normal aerobic muscle metabolism, resulting in an early switch to the anaerobic system. The aerobic metabolism is the system we are dealing with when we speak of aerobic exercise, and it depends on an adequate supply of oxygen, and removal of waste products. If this system becomes overloaded, which it normally would be only in the case of more extreme exertion, there is a switch to the anaerobic metabolism: the anaerobic threshold. (Weight-lifting would be a typical example of anaerobic exercise.) When overdone, this kind of exertion quickly builds up the waste products which cause 'the burn', and delayed and protracted fatigue. The early switch from the aerobic to the anaerobic metabolic system could then account for the delayed and protracted recovery from even minimal exertion which is typical of ME. Exercise, which can improve the strength of muscles in which the aerobic system is functioning properly, becomes damaging to muscles that are overusing the anaerobic, emergency metabolism. This hypothesis could therefore explain why physical exertion, beyond a bare minimum, has been widely observed to make ME symptoms worse.

ME also involves cognitive difficulties and problems in those systems that regulate body temperature and bodily rhythms. This complex web of apparently unrelated symptoms can all be understood as arising from the effects of shape-changes in the red blood cell population. These cause oxygen deprivation in the areas served by the microcirculation (the capillaries) which are particularly sensitive to lack of oxygen: the muscles, the cognitive areas of the brain, and the endocrine system.

However, in contemporary medical literature and medical textbooks, any such symptoms are thought of as circulatory problems – problems with the blood vessels. The connection to shape-changes in the red blood cell population is never made, and treatments that could improve the patient's health by improving the deformability of the red blood cells are not offered. There are, in fact, simple and easily available supplements (listed later in the book) which can improve blood viscosity (the flexibility of the red blood cells), therefore improving the quality of life of many of us who have chronic conditions, including ME. For people trying to figure out how to manage life with ME, this may be the most helpful information in the book.

Now – my part in this!

I have worked in mental health since 1971. My career has included planning the programme and training the staff of a new, purpose-built Humberside Social Services Department day centre for people with mental health problems which opened in 1982; serving as Principal Officer Health for Grimsby and Scunthorpe; then jointly as PO Health for Grimsby and as Humberside Social Services Department's first Information/Policy Officer concerned with HIV. During this period, I also became accredited as a counsellor with the then British Association for Counselling (now renamed the British Association for Counselling and Psychotherapy), and subsequently by the United Kingdom Council for Psychotherapy (UKCP) as a neurolinguistic psychotherapist, and I continue to be accredited by the UKCP.

In April 1986 I acquired what I thought was a mild case of flu after serving as one of four facilitators of a difficult five-day residential group-work course. On the following Monday morning I found that I couldn't do much of anything – just walking across a room meant I had to lie down for ages. If you have ME, or are close to someone who does, you will know what I am talking about. For no particular reason, you find yourself – not ill with anything that you can identify, and not exactly paralysed – but virtually unable to do anything, physical or mental, without suffering extreme exhaustion and mental confusion. Efforts to force oneself beyond this state worsen ones condition, leading to further physical and mental incapacity and pain, with an even longer period of rest needed before recovery. This is frightening and confusing, and you naturally become upset about it. However, it is likely that you have always been pretty healthy and generally able to plough on through the usual illnesses. Therefore, you assume that it's some kind of weird virus and that it will go away in a few days or possibly a couple of weeks, like everything else does. So when it doesn't, you do get increasingly frightened and worried. How long are you going to have to take off work? What do you have to do to get better? Surely you can rise above it and just carry on, like you always have. But the minute you try to do that, you find out that you can't.

As an American who came to England in 1963, I have always been a psychotherapy aficionado, and I have, over the years routinely sought the help of counsellors and psychotherapists when it seemed appropriate. Given this experience in working on my own problems, and my training and experience in working with people who had mental health problems, I felt well qualified to judge whether something that was going on with me had a psychological or psychiatric basis or not. I would have liked nothing better than to know that my current illness would have responded to a psychiatric or psychotherapeutic approach. It was clear to me that it would not.

In my attempts to find out what it could be, I was not encouraged when a search of my symptoms with the library of the local medical school came up with a range of possibilities including MS, leukaemia, and canine distemper! Fortunately, a friend brought me the article about ME which was printed in The Observer during the summer of 1986 [6]. The description fitted my symptoms, and it was a relief to learn that it was not progressive and not fatal. On the contrary, there was the possibility of progress (albeit very protracted) towards recovery. There was no definitive medical test for it, and no medical treatment, but it could be diagnosed through a careful interview, eliciting an account of the symptoms and their variability. At that time, the only suggestion was to rest and to keep exertion within the limits dictated by the illness.

I sent a copy of the article to my doctor, with a letter telling him how relieved I was (and presumed he would be) that I finally had a diagnosis, and wouldn't need to bother him for tests or treatment, as there weren't any. I was very surprised when he arrived at my house in a complete rage that such articles were written, 'giving people ideas', and saying he was sure it was psychiatric. His mood was not improved when I offered to tell him what questions to ask to diagnose depression, and to answer them honestly. He said he could no longer treat me, and referred me to a female colleague in the practice. She very sensibly gave me a thorough examination, listened carefully to my account of my symptoms (and believed what I told her), took routine blood tests to exclude other illnesses, and on that basis accepted a diagnosis of ME. In fact, she proceeded as

Ramsay recommends. She agreed that nothing more would be appropriate, and simply told me to ask her for a sick note when I needed one.

From then on, I treated my illness as a logistical problem, and devised ways to minimise physical exertion while trying to lead as normal a life as possible. These strategies are described in the first part of my story, and summarised in the book's final advice on self-management.

Prompted by the very different practical and emotional responses of my two doctors, I have written about the types of attitude a person with ME is likely to encounter within the medical profession. Your own doctor may or may not be sympathetic and helpful, and you may need some support and help in finding a doctor who is; or dealing with your doctor in a way that can help him or her to cope with the uncertainties and the unpredictable nature of your illness.

An illness which produces a serious degree of incapacity almost immediately, for no clearly understandable medical reason, and which continues for months or years, attracts the interest of medical researchers who genuinely want to understand it and find an effective treatment. However, it is likely to ring alarm bells among both private medical insurers and providers of government incapacity benefits, for whom ME is a very expensive illness. As a result, in these quarters there are strong incentives to give it a psychiatric label, which would assist in invalidating claims on medical insurers and on the U.K. Incapacity Benefit allowances for physical disability.

The classification of ME then becomes of great interest. The symptoms of ME include muscle failure, cognitive difficulties, and endocrine dysfunction, with the added feature of great variability from day to day and even hour to hour. It can sound like raving hypochondria, when in fact it is this overall constellation of symptoms which serves as a defining feature of this illness. However, if, in setting out a list of symptoms purporting to be diagnostic of ME, you include a wider set of unrelated symptoms, including many which are typical of depression, it becomes easier to make a case that the illness is psychiatric. This is evident in the history of the various guidelines, and in the concerted effort, in certain quarters, to rename this illness Chronic Fatigue Syndrome while including unrelated, psychiatric symptoms within that title.

Much of what Dr. Simpson has written in his account of the history of ME and his own work with ME people, as well as his discussion of the various guidelines, gives the reader an insight into this process. My chapters also include references to other detailed accounts of the medical politics which surround this illness.

On the medical side, the challenge is to persuade the medical community that the variable structure and functioning of red blood cells is information which needs to be included within the canon of medical knowledge, so that the many chronic illnesses which are characterised by changes in the shape population of red blood cells can be alleviated to some degree by measures to improve red blood cell deformability.

On the psychiatric side the challenge is how to counteract the power and influence of those psychiatrists who are determined to create and maintain the fiction that ME has no physiological basis. In their view it is entirely the result of 'faulty beliefs', therefore it should be treated by Cognitive Behaviour Therapy. In the context of treating people with ME, the aim of such therapeutic interventions is to persuade them that it is a 'somatoform' psychiatric illness (really all in the mind, but expressed in the form of bodily symptoms). The claim is that the exhaustion experienced by ME sufferers is caused by 'deconditioning', the result of not using muscles, which in turn has been caused by 'over-attention to physical sensations', and that this should be addressed by the coercive use of Graded Exercise Therapy. [7]

This effectively means that many, if not most people who have ME, are offered treatments which will make them worse.

Perhaps you, the reader, may be able and wish to become active in the efforts being made by various groups to get political support for research into the physiological causes of ME, and to counteract the tide of opinion that ME is a 'psychosocial' disorder. We hope this book will provide you with the tools and encouragement to do this.

Nancy Blake

INTRODUCTION

In the preface to the second edition of his book, *Myalgic encephalomyelitis and post-viral fatigue states* (1988), Dr. A.M. Ramsay wrote as follows:

> *The clinical identity of the myalgic encephalomyelitis syndrome rests upon three distinct features, namely:*
>
> 1. *A unique form of muscle fatigability whereby even after a minor degree of physical effort, three, four or five days or longer elapse before full muscle power is restored.*
> 2. *Variability and fluctuations of both symptoms and physical findings in the course of a day; and*
> 3. *An alarming tendency to become chronic.*
>
> *If we take the well-known condition of post-influenzal debility as an example of a post-viral fatigue state, we see that in all these three particulars it constitutes a complete contrast. The wrongful assumption that ME and post viral fatigue states (PVFS) are synonymous, now prevalent in the world literature on the subject, serves to blur the true clinical identity of the myalgic encephalomyelitis syndrome. This can only be remedied when the term PVFS is restored to its rightful context.*

After a general discussion of various outbreaks which were considered to be manifestations of the epidemic form of ME, he discussed the endemic form of ME (p28). He wrote:

> *The patients whom Dr. Scott and I saw came to us in a state of utter despair, their medical advisors finding themselves baffled by a medley of symptoms which they were unable to place into any recognisable category of disease. Without exception, these patients had been referred for consultant opinion and they were generally seen by neurologists who were equally nonplussed, having found no abnormality on physical examination, and with extensive laboratory investigations failing to yield a clue. I must add, however, that in no case had any investigation of the immune system been carried out. Many of the patients were finally referred for psychiatric opinion and it is interesting that four psychiatrists to my knowledge, referred patients back with a note which in essence said, "I do not know what this patient is suffering from, but the case does not come into my field." For the most part, these unfortunate people were finally rejected as hopeless neurotics.*

Dr. Ramsay discussed the multiplicity of symptoms in three groups; muscle phenomena, circulatory impairment and cerebral dysfunction, but no consideration was given to the

9

possibility that muscular and cerebral dysfunction might be other manifestations of circulatory impairment.

Patients who were lucky enough to have a GP who was aware of Dr. Ramsay's work obtained a diagnosis of ME, with normal results from laboratory tests, in terms of Ramsay's concept. An essential feature of such diagnoses was the exclusion of any other possible diagnosis.

Armed with the knowledge that physical activity would exacerbate symptoms, but without any knowledge of the cause or causes of ME, rest became the most obvious form of treatment.

In 1988, an American group introduced the term, "chronic fatigue syndrome" (CFS) to provide a working definition for what had been termed "epidemic neuromyasthenia." The choice of "fatigue" was made without recognition of early reports which had found it impossible to define or to measure fatigue. Unfortunately, the guidelines allowed for the inclusion of many conditions associated with fatigue, and when the criteria were revised in 1994, the new concept was even more inclusive. The resulting confusion as CFS was adopted by other countries, resulted in ME becoming submerged in a sea of other conditions. It is no comfort to learn that many papers on various aspects of CFS have been published, although there is a current attempt to sub-classify CFS patients.

> The category 'Chronic Fatigue Syndrome' was created by making a list of symptoms, not by identifying a specific illness with a specific cause, a specific constellation of symptoms and a specific prognosis. This meant that many conditions, including clinical depression, could fall into this wider category. Research could then be conducted which did not necessarily apply to ME, but by the inclusion of ME into the category 'CFS/ME' or 'ME/CFS', could be alleged to apply to ME. The PACE Trial [8] is the latest example.

To a major extent the situation is exemplified by the book, "The Clinical and Scientific basis of myalgic encephalomyelitis/chronic fatigue syndrome," which was edited by Drs. Hyde, Goldstein and Levine. Contrary to expectations that the book would contain the proceedings of the Cambridge Symposium on ME, it was stated "This text that provides a basis of general information for clinicians and researchers interested in ME/CFS, and was initiated by the Cambridge Easter Symposium on Myalgic Encephalomyelitis /Chronic Fatigue Syndrome."

It is unclear why or how the Cambridge Symposium on ME became a symposium on ME/CFS and it **is a serious omission that there is no record of the proceedings of the symposium.** While Dr. Ramsay was given the title of "Honorary Chairman" of the symposium, only lip-service was paid to his opinions. A major part of the book (sixty-four of seventy-five chapters) was written by Dr. Hyde or by American authors, so from late 1992 when the book was published, ME has struggled against the tide of American-based opinion concerning the importance of CFS.

How did this happen? A Symposium on ME was convened. Papers were presented, discussions held. Someone agreed to publish the proceedings, that is, to collect the papers and records of the discussions, and produce this as a document or book. A book was then published which claimed to 'provide a basis of general information....initiated by the Cambridge Easter Symposium on Myalgic Encephalomyelitis/Chronic Fatigue Syndrome' which produced the 'serious omission' (understatement?) namely 'that there is no record of the proceedings of the symposium.' This sequence of events seems to typify the kind of thing that has happened in the history of ME. (On the other hand, the editors' intention was to provide a powerful scientific case for the fact that what they called ME/CFS is a physiological, not a psychological illness, and they continue to argue for this cause.)

Possibly because of the dominance of CFS and the apparent rejection of the Ramsay concept of ME, the development of various guidelines has not been very helpful. For example, in 1998, the UK Department of Health published a document titled, "Chronic fatigue syndrome/ME," in which it seemed that CFS and ME were synonyms. In 2002, the Chief Medical Officer of the United Kingdom released the report of a CFS/ME Working Group. The report recognised that CFS/ME was a "genuine illness," which indicated that the two terms referred to the same disorder. Subsequently, the Chief Medical Officer invited the Medical Research Council to oversee the research aspects of the report, and that Council established a CFS/ME Research Advisory Board. On December 7, 2002 a CFS/ME Research Strategy was released for public consultation.

Late in 2006, I recognised that if the quality of life of ME sufferers was to be improved, there was an urgent need to separate ME people from the large number of people carrying the CFS label. So I began to work on "Ramsay's Disease."

But early in 2007, a group meeting in Miami (the Name Change Committee) proposed to change CFS to myalgic encephalopathy (ME). In order to avoid early confusion, it was proposed that the disorder should be known as ME/CFS. Subsequently another contributor proposed that the name change should apply only in America. **However, it seems that those involved are determined to compound the confusion created with the introduction of CFS.**

According to Malcolm Hooper [9] this determination was influenced by the response of major medical insurers to the claims for disability resulting from the Lake Tahoe epidemic. (Lake Tahoe is an upmarket resort area where, in the mid 1980's, a large number of young, highly successful and well-off professional people became ill. The media gleefully labelled this 'Yuppie Flu'.) If this illness had been called myalgic encephalomyelitis, it would automatically have been included under the World Health Organisation's categorisation as a neurological disorder. Implicit in that categorisation is that the insurers would have had to pay out for the very high level of physical disability which occurs in ME. However, the U.S. CDC (Center for Disease Control) helpfully gave it the label "Chronic Fatigue Syndrome', CFS. This wider category would allow the possibility of calling it a mental illness, in which case claims for physical disability could be denied. Evidently, large medical insurance companies would be wealthy enough to provide ample rewards for any testimony or evidence which could be offered in support of the mental illness categorisation. In such situations, wealthy corporations are usually able to acquire the 'expert opinions' which support their case. It is important therefore to keep in mind that some of the arguments for the CFS label are founded in the economic interests of insurers, not the health interests of the patients. It is equally possible that the 'evidence-based research' often cited in support of psychiatric bias and psychological treatments may also have been produced with economic incentives.

Therefore the main purpose of writing this book is to ensure that those who have ME, diagnosed in the terms of Ramsay's criteria, should be recognised as having Ramsay's Disease, in order to separate them from ME of CFS origin. It seems fitting to recognise Dr. Ramsay's investigative activities which led to the concept of ME. In addition, the published information will be reviewed to show that the three criteria of Ramsay can be explained in terms of impaired capillary blood flow.

CHAPTER I
- MY WORK WITH ME PEOPLE

In this chapter, Dr. Simpson presents an account of his careful and systematic research which demonstrates that changes in the shape population of red blood cells, which occur during acute phases of ME and not during remissions, directly affect the ability of the red blood cells to deliver oxygen to parts of the body dependent on capillaries. As these include the muscles, the brain, and the endocrine system, this oxygen deprivation can provide an explanation for the constellation of apparently unrelated symptoms present in ME-Ramsay's Disease.

In 1983, through the good offices of Professor Campbell Murdoch, head of the Department of General Practice in the Otago School of Medicine, I met ME patients who were members of the local ME Support Group. It is relevant that in the preceding years I had been writing about the effects of blood viscosity on kidney function and in 1983 (1) we had reported that mice with high levels of protein in their urine also had shape-changed red cells. Such studies were a part of an increasing interest in the flow properties of blood – blood rheology. (2)

So I was very interested in the variability of ME symptoms and the cold hands and feet which immediately stimulated the thought of a blood flow problem.

At that time I had adapted a published technique for filtering blood through polycarbonate filters with 5 micron pores (3), and ethical committee approval was obtained to assess the filterability of the blood of people with ME. Small blood samples, anti-coagulated with EDTA, were obtained from 22 females and 11 males who were considered to be suffering from ME (?ME) and from age and sex matched blood donors. At the lowest filtration pressure there were significant differences between the filtration times of ?ME and blood donor samples, indicating that ME red cells were poorly deformable. Those findings were reported in 1986 (4).

In Lancet 1987 (5), Mukherjee et al reported the presence of abnormally-shaped red cells in 7 ME people after a relapse, noting that the study was stimulated by the 1986 report by Simpson et al. It is noteworthy that the blood samples were anti-coagulated, washed and centrifuged prior to fixation, and although the electron micrographs showed spherical cells with, *"irregular or dimpled surfaces,"* I have never seen similar cells in more than 13,000 samples of immediately fixed blood. However, the authors noted that their results supported the proposal by Simpson et al, that in ME, *"...the microcirculation might be impaired."*

On March 22, 1989, the New Zealand Medical Journal published my paper titled "Nondiscocytic erythrocytes in myalgic encephalo-myelitis."(6) The paper was based on the findings from blood samples from 102 volunteers who believed they suffered from ME and from similar samples from 52 healthy controls and 99 cases of MS which had been selected randomly from a panel of 229 cases in a concurrent study. All blood samples were fixed immediately and underwent the same procedures for preparation for scanning electron microscopy. Following assessment of the micrographs by red cell shape analysis, the results showed that ME blood had the lowest percentage of biconcave discocytes and significantly higher numbers of cup forms than the controls or the MS samples. In addition the MS samples had significantly higher numbers of cells with surface changes than did the control or ME blood samples. It was concluded '…that this type of cell analysis does have the potential to assist in the diagnosis of myalgic encephalomyelitis.'

> So here we have the basis of a blood test which could be a diagnostic tool for ME. Dr. Simpson states later on that red blood cell changes are common in so many other conditions that they cannot be used for the diagnosis of ME. But he agrees that if Dr. Ramsay's criteria are met, including the exclusion of other conditions through standard diagnostic testing, then micrographs of a sample of immediately fixed blood showing a high proportion of non-deformable red cell shapes within the population could serve to support a diagnosis of ME.

Lloyd et al reported in Lancet in July 1989, the results "…of a blinded study of red blood cell morphology by light and scanning electron microscopy in 12 patients with CFS and 10 healthy controls."(7), without reference to my paper published in March. They used the same preparatory techniques as Mukherjee et al had used in their ME study, and found in four cases with CFS (but in no controls) "dimpled spherocytes," and one case showed a slight increase in blood viscosity. However the very low frequency of the "dimpled spherocytes" led to the conclusion that it was unlikely that the red blood cell abnormality, "…is directly associated with the pathophysiology of fatigue in CFS." But because I have never seen such cells in immediately-fixed blood samples, it is likely that the "dimpled spherocytes" are an artefact produced by the preparation techniques.

> The important point here is that the preparation technique used to fix the red blood cells will have an effect on the observations. Samples washed in saline solution will revert to the biconcave discocyte form. Therefore it is necessary to fix the samples immediately to observe the shape changes.

A surprising feature of the scanning electron micrograph in the paper by Lloyd et al and that of Mukherjee et al was that according to the five micron marker, the red cells were less than five microns in diameter.

Later in 1989, the British Journal of Haematology published a paper titled, "Blood from healthy animals and humans contains nondiscocytic erythrocytes," (8) in which I reported that the red blood cells in immediately fixed blood samples could be classified into six different shape classes. That finding led to the development of the technique of red cell shape analysis which has been used to study the red cells from subjects with a wide range of chronic disorders. Because of the immediate fixation, it has been possible to study blood samples from many countries.

14

It needs to be emphasised that there were earlier studies of red cell shape. In the early 1970s there were reports of red cell shape changes in muscular dystrophy. Most studies involved anti-coagulated blood and the results were different from a 1976 study which used immediately fixed blood samples. In that study by Miller et al, (9) it was noted that they were unable to prevent unfixed red cells from changing shape – even in their own plasma in the refrigerator.

A 1977 paper by Markesbery and Butterfield (10) reported that the blood of patients suffering from Huntington's Disease had high values of cup forms (similar to the situation in acute ME). Eight years later, Tanahashi et al used a xenon washout technique to show that Huntington's Disease patients had impaired cerebral blood flow, and the degree of blood flow impairment correlated with cognitive function. But no reference was made to the findings of Markesbery and Butterfield.

Blood samples from children with Down syndrome living in New Zealand (Dunedin, Christchurch), Australia (Toowoomba) and South Africa (Durban) had abnormally high values for flat cells or cup forms. Because of the predictable adverse effect of the shape-changed red cells on blood flow, it is relevant that in 1987, Melamed et al (12) reported that Down syndrome children had impaired cerebral blood flow. The results from the blood samples were presented at a meeting on Downs Syndrome which was held in Darwin in July, 1995. But the idea that impaired blood flow might be important was rejected and the prevailing view was that the only beneficial treatment for Downs children was education.

> How sad, that evidence which could offer hope of a treatment which would help Downs children would simply be rejected! The most well-intentioned people still seem to want to cling to their fixed beliefs in the face of evidence, even to the disadvantage of those they want to help.

As other chronic disorders such as attention deficit and hyperactivity disorder, arthritis, cancer and diabetes for example, also have changed shape populations of red cells it seems that any agent or condition which changes the red cell environment results in changes in the shape populations of red cells. Because of the fact that many other disorders show the sorts of red cell shape changes which occur in ME, the demonstration of changed red cells is not diagnostic for ME. But because the changed red cells contribute to the dysfunctional state of ME, the use of agents to improve red cell deformability becomes a treatment option to eliminate or reduce symptom severity and to improve the quality of life of sufferers.

At the Cambridge Symposium in 1990, I presented a paper titled, "The role of nondiscocytic erythrocytes in the pathogenesis of myalgic encephalomyelitis," but when it was published in Hyde's book in 1992, the title had had '/chronic fatigue syndrome' added at the end. The paper was based on the findings from red cell shape analysis of immediately fixed blood samples from 39 males and 60 females, "...*who suffered from chronic tiredness and easy fatigability,*" because of their ME. The results were very similar to those of the 102 cases which had been published in 1989.

In the abstracts of the "Summerland ME/CFS Seminar," held in Lismore, NSW on Sept.21-22, 1991, Dr. Ian Buttfield wrote about "Red blood cells – Dr. Tarpon (sic) Mukherjee". He noted that with the use of a new, powerful electron microscope, an attempt would be made to determine if the abnormal red cells could be used as a diagnostic test. Then he discussed the difficulties in obtaining a diagnostic test. No mention was made of my 1986 or 1989 papers. It was proposed that, *"A pilot study of the abnormal red cells in ME will commence in Adelaide in May 1992 and could be finished in 4 or 5 months."* I have not been able to find anything published about the pilot study, but by mid-1992 I would have assessed more than 400 ME blood samples.

This is one of many examples of the apparent invisibility of Dr. Simpson's extensive number of publications. One wonders how much knowledge is lost, or experiments repeated, or sound ideas simply ignored, because of the failure of communication from one journal to another, or the failure of researchers to make a thorough search for papers relevant to the work they are proposing to do. There must be a lot of people out there re-inventing the wheel. And undoubtedly, research, however conscientiously conducted, will tend to get brushed aside if it contradicts currently fashionable concepts. There is a detailed analysis of this process (citation bias) in [10]

During the seminar, Dr. Buttfield was asked, "What are your personal views on a lack of oxygen in tissue?" He replied, "I believe that ME is primarily related to problems in the brain, and one part of that may well be a lack of oxygen in the tissues, including the brain." His reply makes it clear that he was not associating shape-changed red cells with oxygen delivery.

A paper titled, "Idiopathic chronic fatigue. A primary disorder," was published in 1990, in New Jersey Medicine. I submitted a reply, which was accepted and published in March 1992, with the changed title, "Chronic tiredness and idiopathic chronic fatigue – a connection?" (13) Not only was there a short editorial comment, but also the published paper included beautifully presented plates which clearly identified the different red cell shapes, except for early and late cup forms. In the text it was suggested

> *...that subjects with the symptom of tiredness and high percentages of nondiscocytic cells in their blood, would have smaller-than-usual capillaries; i.e. those with mean capillary diameter falling within the first quartile of a size distribution. Subjects with this characteristic would always be at risk of red-cell-shape-related impairment of capillary blood flow.*

Such a proposal could explain in part, why some people recover from a viral infection within one or two weeks, while others become chronically unwell and develop ME. While both groups will respond to a viral infection with shape-changed red cells, it seems that in those with ME some other factor is "switched" on, and the shape-changed red cells persist until the factor is "switched" off resulting in a period of remission. In addition, the concept of smaller-than-usual capillaries could explain the great variability in presenting symptoms of ME people, which could represent the effects of randomly distributed clusters of small capillaries.

In developing the concept that the major symptom of ME is chronic tiredness, it seems relevant to draw attention to a significant, but seldom quoted paper titled, "The clinical significance of tiredness," by Dr. Geoffrey Ffrench, published in 1960 (14). The paper was based upon data that related to 105 cases with a primary complaint of tiredness which had been extracted from almost 1200 consecutive cases. In the summary it was stated,

> These (data) have been analysed and the relation of tiredness to specific conditions defined, particularly the predominance of tiredness as a symptom of physical rather than neurotic disorder. An attempt has been made to integrate the physiological and psychological processes which may take part in the production of this symptom, with particular reference to disorders of the endocrine, genito-urinary and haemopoietic systems in relation to specific processes of metabolism.

The author noted

> Tiredness is a "whole" symptom. It is felt throughout the patient's body and is not confined to regions, anatomic structures or specific physiological functions, but rather it emanates from the natural whole of the body and mind.

It was concluded, "There is no doubt that oxygen lack is the first cause of tissue cell exhaustion, which is manifested early by clinical tiredness."

This statement is wholly compatible with Simpson's Axiom, **"Persistently impaired capillary blood flow is absolutely incompatible with normal tissue function."** According to Ffrench, the practical application of his study was

> ...that when a spontaneous complaint of tiredness, lassitude, lack of drive or exhaustion is made, careful inquiry and examination must be undertaken before consigning the case to what has been described as the clinical rubbish basket of neurotic ill-health.

Note the similarity of the idea of "neurotic ill-health" to the outcome of many people with ME in their search for a sympathetic physician.

> Ffrench warns against consigning the patient complaining of tiredness to 'the clinical rubbish basket of neurotic ill health.' Yet, that is the experience of many of us, and the Wessely group are now working hard to have what they call CFS/ME classified in a new psychiatric category in DSM-5, the forthcoming edition of the American Diagnostic and Statistical Manual: 'Somatoform Symptom Disorder' (the posh name for 'it's all in your head') – which seems likely to become the new 'clinical rubbish basket'.
>
> Ffrench's injunction that 'careful enquiry and examination must be undertaken' seems also to suggest respectful enquiry – which could elicit the difference between the highly motivated person with ME who attempts a task and finds it impossible to carry on, and then gets upset, as against the person burdened with the sadness and apathy of depression, who when urged to attempt a task, may find their mood improved by the effort.

The most controversial aspect of "chronic fatigue syndrome," relates to the term "fatigue" and much has been written about the topic. In a 1984 paper titled, "Malaise and fatigue," (15) Sir John Ellis noted that although malaise and fatigue are terms which recur through medical textbooks,

> ...patients hardly ever use these terms. They complain of being tired and not feeling well. When asked to be more precise, they say they are knackered, bushed,

beat, washed out, drained or utterly exhausted (all of which may or may not mean the same thing).

It could be important that the medical use of the term fatigue seems not to recognise dictionary definitions where fatigue is the consequence of long-continued exertion.

This diversion into the significance of tiredness relates to a study of the effects of trigger-finger fatigue on red cell shape in ME people and healthy controls. (16) The primary observation was a war time experience of seeing who could pull a revolver trigger for the most times. The onset of trigger finger fatigue was very strange, as although you willed your finger to pull the trigger, it remained inactive. On the basis that the muscle mass of the trigger finger was too small to induce a relapse in ME people, in 1993, an application was made for ethical approval of a study in which ME people would provide blood samples before and after pulling the trigger of an antique revolver. However, the local ethics committee ruled that, **"...as myalgic encephalomyelitis was an indefinable disorder, it was not permissible to use myalgic encephalomyelitis in the title of the study." Approval was granted when ME was replaced by, "...those suffering from chronic tiredness."**

> This is a striking example of the need for a clearly defined and generally accepted name for this illness. If 'Ramsay's Disease (ME)' was in the title of every research paper concerning ME, and such research excluded all the other conditions which can be included under the umbrella of CFS and all its variants, it would become much easier to provide proof of the physiological nature of this illness.

The timing of the study related to a weekend, residential meeting of members of ME Support Groups and it eventually involved 69 ME volunteers and 72 healthy controls. Three-drop samples of immediately fixed blood were obtained before commencement of trigger pulling and immediately after the onset of trigger finger fatigue. The elapsed time and the number of trigger pulls were recorded. After a rest period of 5 minutes, the test and blood sampling was repeated. Blood samples were prepared for scanning electron microscopy and the resulting micrographs were subjected to red cell shape analysis. Healthy controls comprised people in non-sedentary occupations such as teachers, nurses, and members of the fire service, police force or army.

The results showed that in the pre-trigger-pulling samples, the red cell shape populations of ME people were significantly different from those of the controls. ME people had significantly fewer trigger pulls with a shorter time until the onset of muscle fatigue. After the second trigger pull, the differences were greater. It was concluded that,

> *...the association of shape-transformed red cells and impaired muscle function in subjects suffering from chronic tiredness draws attention to the pathogenic potential of nondiscocytic erythrocytes. The results of this study indicate that therapeutic measures aimed at the restoration of normal red cell flexibility could have benefits for those suffering from persisting tiredness.*

This simple study, which linked low-level muscle activity to changes in the shape populations of red cells, provides a basis for understanding the relationship between physical activity and relapses in ME. It would be reasonable to propose that the use of larger muscles would induce greater degrees of change in red cell shape, with a corresponding adverse effect on the flow properties of blood. This would explain the results from SPECT scans carried out by Dr. Goldstein, in California, on a patient who came to Dunedin for a blood test. She gave me the SPECT scans which showed that a pre-exercise scan had reduced cerebral blood flow which was much worse in a post-exercise scan.

The results from the trigger-pulling study were presented at the International CFS/ME Research Conference, in Albany, NY, on October 4. 1992. During lunch break on that day I was approached by a member of a support group who asked if I would meet with other sufferers at the conclusion of the meeting. As a result, notices went up to say that Dr. Simpson would meet with sufferers at 4.30 pm, in a named room. At the appointed time, 25 people arrived, and after a question and answer session there was a vigorous discussion. This went on until 6 pm when a janitor arrived and asked that the room be vacated. Group discussions continued as they walked away from the room. There was a marked difference in the ambience of the meeting when compared to that of the Cambridge Symposium, and I was left with the feeling that those involved considered CFS/ME an interesting research topic, with little evident sympathy or empathy for sufferers, and some of the post-presentation discussions were very heated. The proceedings of the meeting were to be published in the Journal of Infectious Diseases, but **the editor would not accept the idea that red cells changed shape,** and I was requested to re-write. After three revisions were rejected, I withdrew the paper, so there is no record that I participated in the meeting.

Note the phrase 'the editor would not accept the **idea** that red cells changed shape.' But Dr Simpson has provided **evidence**, slides taken using electron microscopy, that they do change shape - that the populations of red blood cells in people who have ME have a much increased proportion of irregularly shaped red blood cells. This, therefore, is 'information', not 'an idea'. Yet the editor can simply reject this information because he – what? Hasn't read the research? Doesn't want to believe it? It doesn't fit with what he has learned? What? This illustrates the fact that scientists do not always respond in an objective, dispassionate manner to facts which conflict with their beliefs. Citation bias [10], one aspect of which is ignoring published work which conflicts with accepted ideas, is taken a step further when such work is not even published.

In the book edited by Hyde, Goldstein and Levine, there were only two references to the remissions experienced by ME people. On page 105, Dr. P. Snow noted, *"The disease over the years had demonstrated its chronic remitting and relapsing nature,"* and on page 530, Dr. Loblay, in a chapter on "Pathogenesis," stated, *"the fluctuating course, both short term and long-term, the occurrence of spontaneous remissions, (occasionally full recovery) even after prolonged illness."* Having met ME people who were in remission for up to three days, one case in particular is of interest. A young woman brought a blood sample to my office about 9 am one morning. On inspecting the application form, I noticed that she had declared that she was "well", and I pointed out that if she was well then the sample would probably have normal results. About 4 pm on the same day, she arrived with another sample as she had "crashed" about 3.30, and was severely unwell. When the samples were eventually assessed, they showed the first sample as normal and the second sample as being grossly abnormal.

That case stimulated a study of remissions in thirty-two females and eleven males who had had a physician's diagnosis of ME at least two years previously. At baseline and at 4-weekly-intervals for forty weeks, we met to obtain blood samples and to complete a questionnaire concerning their symptom severity and wellbeing. The results showed that at one extreme there were five women who had abnormal blood results in all eleven blood samples, while at the other extreme was one woman who had normal blood tests in six of her eleven samples. The most frequent result was to have two periods of remission with normal blood tests, during the forty weeks. As remissions could have occurred at other times, this was a minimal situation, and indicated that remissions were not rare events.

The results from the trigger-pulling study were underscored by the experience of a high school girl who presented a record of her personal experience at a school Science Fair. (17)

In addition to fixing a blood sample before and after trigger pulling, part of the blood sample was added to 5ml of sterile saline for five minutes before the red cells were removed and fixed. She followed the usual procedures for red cell preparation, sputter coating and scanning electron microscopy, and red cell shape analysis. In the pre-trigger pulling sample, there were 67.9% discoid cells and 10.6% cells with altered margins (echinocytes). The onset of fatigue occurred after thirty-five seconds and during that time the discoid cells had fallen to 56.4% while cells with altered margins had increased to 30.4%. But after five minutes in saline, the 67.9% discoid cells had increased to 82.1%, and the cells with altered margins had fallen to 0.9% in the pre-trigger-pulling sample. In the post trigger-pulling sample the 56.8% discoid cells had increased to 85% and cells with altered margins had fallen to 0.4%.

This simple study showed that in a healthy subject, the red cell shape populations may change quickly and dramatically. Furthermore, exposure to a saline solution caused red cells to transform towards the textbook concept of red cell shape. It was concluded, ***"These observations highlight the existence of conflict between concepts of red cell shape based on observations of immediately-fixed red cells, and the observations on cells which had been washed and manipulated before fixation."*** Although this was the first report of saline-induced changes in red cell shape, the judges failed to recognise the implications of the finding.

Three physicians provided immediately-fixed blood samples prior to, and after they had completed running a marathon. In all three post-race samples, there were abnormally high numbers of cup forms (stomatocytes) with the lowest number associated with a running time of two hours thirty minutes, and the highest number associated with a race time of four hours ten minutes. Such observations reinforce the idea that red cell shape is a dynamic factor. As red cells lose the nucleus when they leave the bone marrow, they may lack the capacity for independent existence and are at the mercy of their environment.

In order to obtain from general practitioners an assessment of the usefulness of the results from red cell shape analysis in managing ME patients, an anonymous questionnaire was sent to twenty-four general practitioners who had sent blood samples from ME patients between 1/7/93 and 31/12/93. All questionnaires were returned and 78% considered the results from red cell shape analysis to be helpful or very helpful, and the results influenced decisions on diagnosis and treatment in 74% of cases. Almost all respondents (96%) considered the results were useful for explanations to patients.

According to my daily diary, between October 1993 and December 2000, I visited and spoke to two hundred seventy-four Support Groups, most of which were ME, in seven countries. Between July 1998 and December 2000, thirty-five of the meetings were with either ME/Fibromyalgia or Fibromyalgia groups. Even though no audience numbers were recorded for thirteen meetings, the audiences totalled eight thousand nine hundred and fifty people. The details of those visits are as follows: Australia, twenty-three groups mainly on the east coast; Canada, seventy-six groups from St Johns in Newfoundland to Terrace and Fort St. John in northern British Columbia; Ireland, two groups, Belfast and Dublin; New Zealand, ten groups in both North and South Islands; South Africa, eight groups from Nelsprit in the north to Capetown in the south; United Kingdom, ninety-eight groups from Lands End to Glasgow; USA, fifty-three groups scattered across the continent. Although I paid my own travel costs, most of the expense was recovered by collections or admission charges. In most cases I was privileged to be billeted with a member of the group being visited.

The large number of groups visited in England reflects the efficiency of rail travel. During some visits I would speak to a group at 10.30, travel one-hundred miles by rail, speak again at 2.30, catch another train and speak again at 7.30 pm. Such visits were made possible by the dedication of group leaders who would provide me with a speaking programme with details of the trains I had to catch.

As a result of these meetings with ME people, and prolonged question and answer sessions, I learned a great deal about ME and how it affected the quality of life. When time allowed, I was happy to visit "shut-ins", i.e. people who were so unwell they were housebound. During such visits I made a point of emphasising the need for some level of physical activity.

Physical activity in a healthy person improves blood viscosity by improving the deformability (flexibility) of the red blood cells. A person who has ME can benefit from this effect, but will be made worse if exercise exceeds the very narrow limits before failure of oxygen delivery results in a transition from the aerobic to the anaerobic muscle metabolism. For this reason, Dr. Simpson points out the potential benefit of 'some level of physical activity' to the bedbound and mostly immobile patient, and he is careful to specify that this must be undertaken only when the patient feels up to it.

This fits with the concept of 'pacing' of activity as controlled by the patient which many patients find beneficial. It is quite different from a prescription of Graded Exercise Therapy determined by a set program, underpinned by a belief that the patient's problem is psychological, and, sometimes accompanied by a basically hostile and punitive attitude on the part of the professionals involved.

Perhaps the most important aspect of the meetings was the collection of blood samples, and in many cases, during subsequent visits it was possible to discuss the implications of the results from their blood samples.

During my third visit to Canada, on December 5, 1996, I spoke to the ME Support Group in Victoria, British Columbia. At the completion of question time, I was approached by Dr. Abram Hoffer, editor of the Journal of Orthomolecular Medicine, who invited me to submit a paper based upon the lecture he had just heard. So in the middle of 1997, the paper was published under the title, "Myalgic encephalomyelitis (ME): a haemorheological disorder manifested as impaired capillary blood flow." (18) The paper concluded,

> *The main message in this paper is that you will feel only as well as your capillaries deliver oxygen and nutrient to your tissues. Therefore, when altered blood rheology impairs capillary blood flow, there will be an adverse effect on wellbeing.*

Finally,

> *My interest in ME is based solely upon a desire to help a section of the community who suffer from a debilitating illness which has yet to gain acceptance from the medical community. At the risk of being considered irrational about the biological importance of normal capillary blood flow, I can point with satisfaction to the many ME patients who have benefited from treatment with haemorheological agents.*

Later in 1997 Dr. Hoffer accepted and published a paper titled, "The results from red cell shape analyses of blood samples from members of myalgic encephalomyelitis organisations in four countries."(19)

The paper summarised the results obtained from two thousand one hundred and seventy eight blood samples contributed from Australia (ten groups); England (twenty-seven groups); New Zealand (four groups) and South Africa (six groups). The range of ages of those providing blood samples was similar for all countries – five to sixty-five years, and apart from New Zealand, the average age was about forty-four years. In contrast, the New Zealand average ages were 32.6 years for males and 37.7 years for females.

Because of the known effect of age on red cell shape, the results from sixty-three cases (New Zealand, twenty-four, Australia, twenty-nine, England ten) who were seventy years or older were excluded from the analysis.

The most frequent change in the shape populations of red cells was an increase in flat cells, and this value was highest in English samples. In agreement with the recognised fluctuation of symptoms, an average of about 12% of samples had no abnormal values. The range of such events was from 2% (in English samples) to about 22% (in Australian samples).

An interesting aspect of this blood testing was that prior to 1990, blood samples from ME people were marked by increased cup forms which were considered the marker for acute ME. But between 1990 and 1992 there was a change toward high values for flat cells (a marker for chronic ME) with only about 5% of cases having high values for cup forms.

When dealing with American samples, a major problem arose from their use of diagnostic terms. Because it was not possible to decide on the relationship of CFS, or CFS/CFIDS or CFIDS/CFS/FM to ME, the results from American samples were published in 2001, in a paper titled, "Red blood cell shape, symptoms and reportedly helpful treatments in Americans with chronic disorders."(20) A total of six-hundred thirty two blood samples in seven different categories were assessed. The average ages were higher than those in the ME report and ranged from forty-six years to 50.2 years. In all categories, the major change was a high value for flat cells which ranged from73.3% to 79.4%, so there is little doubt that impaired capillary blood flow would be a contributing factor in the chronic disorders.

> At this point, we begin to see the effects of the re-labelling of ME (Myalgic Encephalomyelitis) as CFS (Chronic Fatigue Syndrome), CFIDS (Chronic Fatigue Immune Deficiency Syndrome), FM (Fibromyalgia). As mentioned previously, Professor Malcolm Hooper's document, entitled 'Corporate Collusion?' explains the influence of the psychiatric lobby on various groups brought together for the purpose of developing guidelines for a diagnosis of what in the U.K. is now called CFS/ME. 'Post-exercise malaise' is not even included as a defining symptom in the Oxford Criteria and it has been said that people who experience this symptom have been eliminated from the patient samples for their research into CFS/ME. This would have the effect of specifically excluding anyone suffering from ME from the research cohort, although they will then apply the treatments researched in this way to patients who do have ME. For a detailed account of this process, see [11]

The problem of diagnostic terms arose again in Alberta, Canada, with only 44 of 238 samples labelled as ME, while 66 were labelled CFS and 28 had composite names. In addition 103 were labelled as fibromyalgia. Only 35 of the participants were males. The samples were obtained during snowy weather from Calgary, Camrose, Edmonton, Grand Prairie, Lethbridge, Medicine Hat and Red Deer. In each diagnostic category from all communities, the average ages were very variable, ranging from a 30-year-old female in Camrose to two sixty-year-olds in Red Deer. The most common finding in the red cell shape data was high values for flat cells in all disease categories which ranged from 82.3% in a sample from a Camrose male with fibromyalgia to 67.8% in a male in Edmonton with CFS.

It was suggested that because of the variety of diagnoses quoted, ME, CFIDS, FM, CFS, CFS/FM and CFS/ME, there was an urgent need to introduce a greater degree of uniformity in naming the condition.

It is worth noting that in the preparation of the various guidelines which have been developed to aid the management of ME/CFS, there is no recognition of or reference to my work. It seems safer simply to ignore new information than to attempt to incorporate that information into a fallacious concept. So at this time, none of the "guidelines" provides a basis for understanding the nature of remissions which were a key factor in Ramsay's concepts of ME. It would be very difficult to imagine a disease process caused by a persistent viral infection or a persisting immunological aberration, which allowed a return to "normality" for hours, days or weeks.

My last attempt to interest physicians in the pathogenic role of blood rheology in ME was a paper in the December issue, 2002, of the New Zealand Family Physician, titled, "On the pathophysiology of ME/CFS."(21) However, the paper failed to produce any response. So although I continued to evaluate blood samples up to September 2003, I felt that the authorities were not being convinced, and it made no sense to continue to expend my savings, so I closed down.

> The question of how scientific information can become accepted as fact within the body of medical knowledge and within the wider public domain is central to the whole issue of ME. Blood rheology is simply ignored in medical literature, despite many, many accounts of symptoms, and the effects of various medical interventions, which are coded as 'not understood', but which can clearly be explained by reference to the research by rheologists. And in the meantime, the psychiatric community have managed to get the psychosocial model of ME accepted as 'scientific fact' simply by ignoring and deleting reference to the thousands of research papers demonstrating physical effects. These are both effects of **citation bias.** [10]

Chapter I References

1. Simpson LO, Shand BI, Olds RJ. Echinocytes in the blood of hyperproteinemic mice with proteinuria. Is the effect of such cells on blood viscosity the cause of the proteinuria? British Journal of Experimental Pathology 1983; 64:594-8.
2. Dintenfass L. Rheology of blood in diagnostic and preventive medicine. Butterworths, London, 1976.
3. Reid HL, Barnes AJ, Lock PJ, et al. A simple method for measuring erythrocyte deformability. Journal of Clinical Pathology 1976; 29; 855-8.
4. Simpson LO, Shand BI, Olds RJ. Blood rheology and myalgic encephalomyelitis: a pilot study. Pathology 1986; 18:190-2.
5. Mukherjee TM, Smith K, Maros K. Abnormal red cell morphology in myalgic encephalomyelitis. (Letter) Lancet 1987; 2:328-9.
6. Simpson LO. Nondiscocytic erythrocytes in myalgic encephalomyelitis. New Zealand Medical Journal 1989; 102:106-7.
7. Lloyd A, Wakefield D, Smith L, et al. Red cell morphology in chronic fatigue syndrome. (Letter) Lancet 1989; 2:217.
8. Simpson LO. Blood from healthy animals and humans contains nondiscocytic erythrocytes. British Journal of Haematology 1989; 73:561-4.
9. Miller SE, Roses AD, Appel SH. Scanning electron microscopy studies in muscular dystrophy. Archives of Neurology 1976; 33:172-4.
10. Markesbery WR, Butterfield DA. A scanning electron microscope study of erythrocytes in Huntington's Disease. Biochemical and Biophysical Research Communications 1977; 78:560-4.

11. Tanahashi N, Meyer JS, Ishikawa Y, et al. Cerebral blood flow and cognitive testing correlate in Huntington's Disease. Archives of Neurology 1985; 42:1167-75.
12. Melamed E, Mildworf B, Sharav T, et al. Regional cerebral blood flow in Down's Syndrome. Annals of Neurology 1987; 22:275-8
13. Simpson LO. Chronic tiredness and idiopathic chronic fatigue – a connection? New Jersey Medicine 1992; 89:211-6.
14. Ffrench G. The clinical significance of tiredness. Canadian Medical Association Journal 1960; 80:665-71.
15. Ellis J. Malaise and fatigue. British Journal of Hospital Medicine 1984;32:312-4.
16. Simpson LO, Murdoch JC, Herbison GP. Red cell shape changes following trigger finger fatigue in subjects with chronic tiredness and controls. New Zealand Medical Journal 1993; 106:104-7.
17. Simpson LO. Red cell shape. (Letter) New Zealand Medical Journal 1993; 106:531.
18. Simpson LO. Myalgic encephalomyelitis (ME): a haemorheological disorder manifested as impaired capillary blood flow. Journal of Orthomolecular Medicine 1997; 12:69-76.
19. Simpson LO, Herbison GP. The results from red cell shape analysis of blood samples from members of myalgic encephalomyelitis organisations in four countries. Journal of Orthomolecular Medicine 1997; 12:221-6.
20. Simpson LO, O'Neill DJ. Red blood cell shape, symptoms and reportedly helpful treatments in Americans with chronic disorders. Journal of Orthomolecular Medicine 2001; 16:157-65.
21. Simpson LO. On the pathophysiology of ME/CFS. New Zealand Family Physician 2002; 29:426-8.

The events immediately before and after I became ill in April, 1986 are described in the Explanation of The Book. It may make the rest of my story more coherent if I give a timeline of events in my life.

Life before ME

1957   Graduated from Boston University cum laude in Romance Languages and Literature, with a minor in Philosophy/ Psychology.

1957-61   Employed as a technical secretary at Massachusetts Institute of Technology. My job was mainly typing up papers for publication in scientific journals and technical textbooks. Two years in the Department of Mathematics, subsequently in the Chemistry Department.

1961   Married Postdoctoral student Tony Blake.

1963   March – August: Tony and I drove from Boston to Buenos Aires, via Mexico, Central America, Colombia, Ecuador, Peru, Bolivia and Argentina. We embarked on a boat trip from Buenos Aires to Portugal, drove through Spain and France to the U.K., arriving in August.

1963   September: Came to Hull, where Tony took up post as Lecturer in Chemistry. We settled down in an old cottage in the tiny village of Aike 18 miles from Hull. I worked as a secretary in the Market Research Department at Reckitt and Colman until we started our family.

1964   Son Andrew born 18 July, daughter Julie 16 November 1965.

1968-72   Taught Adult Education classes in Driffield and Scarborough.

1969-71   Completed Diploma in the Teaching of Adults, and Graduate Diploma in Social Administration at the University of Hull.

1971-80   I worked at Pashby House, a Day Hospital for people with mental health problems, run jointly by the NHS and the Social Services Department.

1980-81   I did a diploma in Applied Social Studies, completed requirements for the Certificate of Qualification in Social Work, University of Leeds.

1981   April: On placement with the Ventura County Mental Health Services, California, U.S.A. This is where I first heard about John Grinder and Richard Bandler's seminars in neurolinguistic programming – NLP.

LESLIE O. SIMPSON & NANCY BLAKE

1981-83   Intensive-Care Social Worker at the East Hull Social Services Department, specialising in complex, 'fat-file' cases.

1983-86   Officer in Charge, Brunswick Avenue Centre, Hull. This was a purpose-built day centre for people with mental health problems.

1985   Moved to Hull, to a bigger house in Park Avenue.

Life with ME

1986   April-August: Off sick with ME

1986-87   Principal Officer for Health Grimsby and Scunthorpe, covering another worker's maternity leave.

1987   Continued as Principal Officer for Health Grimsby, half-time; half-time working as the department's first Information/Policy Officer for HIV.

1986-87   Served on working party setting out plans for mental health services in the 1990's. Helped present the report, 'Well Into the Future' to the Humberside County Council, who granted £1million to carry out the proposals.

1988-89   Reorganisation of the Social Services Department; took the only post offered, as Senior Social Worker, Castle Hill Hospital

1989   Retired from the Social Services Department.

1988-89   Houses: In 1988, made a formal separation agreement with my husband which enabled me to purchase four small houses in the wrong end of town and undertake an unsuccessful career as a landlady.

1990's   NLP: Completed Practitioner Course in 1990, Human Design Engineering 1993, Master Practitioner, 1994.

1996   Joined the Executive Committee of the then Psychotherapy and Counselling Section of the Association for NLP (ANLP PCS). Post of Chair 1997-1999. I was able to carry out this role only because Russ Meyer had become a colleague, and did most of the driving in our trips to London. Another bit of well-timed good fortune!

1986-   Psychotherapy Began private practice in 1986, BAC Accredited 1987, UKCP Registered, then Accredited from 1995 to the present.

1987-   Teaching piano Began teaching piano informally, mainly adult beginners, non-exam. Including teaching at a local private primary school from 2008, I now have about 20 pupils.

Current   Sharing a house with my friend, Sue and her son, Ethan, teaching piano, doing psychotherapy, writing this.

Looking back, it seems as though my getting ill was the catalyst for many other changes in my life. I gradually moved out of the marital home, eventually retired from my job, got my ears pierced and started singing at The Adelphi, a local club where my son and his friend had initiated an amateur night. I took a trip through the south of England, busking with a friend. (With my wheelchair and my dog, and my Peavey amp and microphone, I must have looked the part.) In the 1988 property frenzy, I managed to buy four small, dilapidated houses at the wrong end of town and discovered that being a landlady was an extremely stressful occupation, not to be undertaken without building and business management skills. So not a good idea if you've got ME.

It was a hectic time. This sounds light-hearted and rather flippant. Actually, I was living as people do when reminded that health, and life, can come to an end – 'doing the things you've always wanted to do' suddenly becomes an urgent matter, urgent to the point of desperation. So I became, simultaneously, an invalid and an adventuress.

Having ME did simplify some of my decisions. Previously I had been caught up in a chaotic network of obligations. On the one hand were the things I felt obliged to do for other people and on the other, the things I felt obliged to do because they were good for you. For example, I had got myself into a pattern of weekly evening visits to people who I thought were in need, which I felt obliged to maintain despite my full-time job and family responsibilities. These visits occupied four nights a week and this had become part of the unsustainable overload of activities in my life. Post ME, if someone wanted to see me, they would have to become the visitor. Interestingly, the people I had so assiduously visited didn't return the favour. (Maybe they were as relieved as I was!)

Similarly, physical activities for their own sake were right off the list. Before ME, I used to run rather than walk (but drive rather than run!) and I adored swimming and horseback riding. After we moved into the city I liked to get out for walks in the country. Now I didn't have to debate whether I had the time or energy to do those things. I had to debate how long I would have to rest before being able to put on the next item of clothing during the lengthy and exhausting process of getting dressed; or deliberate over how long I could put off undertaking the long walk to the toilet.

People who believe that the illnesses we get, and the accidents we have, teach us something about our lives are probably not that far wrong. We know that long-term stress contributes to heart disease and stroke, and it depresses the immune system thereby rendering us vulnerable to whatever illnesses are going around. We know that lifestyle issues such as drinking, smoking, and overeating have direct connections to health problems. Too often, as in the case of the person diagnosed with lung cancer who finally decides to stop smoking, the 'Lesson', if we want to call it that, gets learned too late. It is true that for years, my experience of trying to get through all the physical and emotional tasks of daily living had made me feel as though I was being squeezed through a tube, like toothpaste. It is true that becoming physically 'wiped out' by ME forced a definite limit on the sorts of things that I was able to do, simplifying a life-pattern that had become impossible to sustain.

It is interesting that many people who have ME are described, pre-illness, as energetic, ambitious, very active people. In the efforts to classify ME a psychiatric problem, these personal qualities are re-labelled as pathological. In a successful individual who remained healthy, these same qualities would be regarded as positive attributes contributing to their success.

In describing the overloaded life I was leading before I got ill, I may seem to be playing into the hands of those who want to label us as suffering from a purely psychosocial disorder. On the contrary, I am making the point that generally speaking people who become ill with ME do not have the type of personality likely to 'give in' to an illness, let alone enjoy it. It may be that our enthusiasm, commitment to our professions, and possibly over-energetic lifestyles leave us vulnerable to whatever agent or agents it is that produces the physiological dysfunctions we experience (which, as Dr. Simpson shows, are manifested through the effects of stiffened red blood cells). And it is those same personal qualities which produce the courageous determination to persist, despite illness, that lead us to make efforts that in so many cases intensify the symptoms and increase the level and duration of our disability. My point is that 'treatments' based on the presupposition that physical exertion should be imposed on us merely serve to add injury to insult.

The First Signs of Becoming Ill

In 1981, I was commuting weekly to Leeds to take the Diploma in Applied Social Studies, which would also give me the Certificate of Qualification in Social Work. I had been advised that this qualification would be essential if I were to progress in my career, and had successfully applied for secondment.

We were living in Aike which was a tiny village (thirteen houses) when we first moved there. It was eighteen miles from Hull where Tony was a lecturer in the Department of Chemistry at the University of Hull and eight miles from Beverley (the nearest reasonably-sized town). The bus stop was three miles away.

We had two ponies, and one of my jobs each weekend, in addition to catching up with the laundry and baking bread for the family, was bringing their week's supply of hay down from a neighbouring farm. This involved transporting four heavy bales in a wheelbarrow: an effort that stretched me to the limit of my physical endurance.

I drove the sixty miles to Leeds each Sunday night, returning on Friday, in a fairly ancient Ford. My extra-curricular activities included the occasional disco dance, horse riding, and folk-dancing. All in all, not a restful existence!

In 1981, during the Easter break, I suffered my first bout of serious fatigue, which necessitated my spending virtually the entire two weeks unable to do more than lie about. However I did recover sufficiently to get back to Leeds and complete the course successfully.

After the course, the Social Services Department deployed me away from Pashby House to the post as Intensive Care Social Worker. This was a thoroughly enjoyable job designed to relieve social workers of their most demanding, 'fat-file' cases. I was to have a small case-load of these clients in order to work with them intensively, in the hope that they could be returned to their social-worker in a much more manageable state. It was a no-lose situation: these cases were regarded as hopeless, so if you didn't get anywhere, no one had expected you could, and if you did get somewhere, you were a miracle-worker. The clients were fascinating, and of course, if you had all the time in the world and the freedom to help in whatever way you saw fit, progress was possible. As several of the cases were complicated by psychiatric problems, this involved close liaison with the psychiatrist who served the area. We formed a mutually respectful collaboration in those cases.

However, this rewarding period was interrupted for a few weeks after a Christmas break (1982) when I had succumbed to a mild flu, and didn't seem to get better. My GP told me that it was important to rest, and my sick notes labelled my condition 'post-viral debilitation'. On the fifth week, he wrote 'post-viral depression'. With the hint that it might be labelled something psychiatric, I decided it must be time to get back to work, which I found myself able to do. This pattern of recovery would fit with Ramsey's definition of Post-Viral Fatigue Syndrome.

After a year, the Department started advertising posts for the new, purpose-built centre for people with mental health problems, as part of the program of closure of the big mental hospitals and transfer of mental health care from the NHS to the Social Services. I got the post of Manager. For four years, I worked hard at this, despite various difficulties with the Social Services Department.

We had a very interesting group of clients who came for a weekly evening group-therapy session. They were mature, intelligent professionals and well able to make life challenging for their group leader.

In April 1986, a few months after we had moved from Aike to Park Avenue in Hull, one of these clients stopped me as I was leaving after the group, to ask how on earth I managed to keep myself OK, in the context of dealing with all this human distress. I explained cheerfully that if you knew that you were helping people, it did give you the extra energy to go on. That was the last conversation I had with him, until years later.

The following week, I was assisting at a residential group-work week which turned out to be particularly difficult, and by the end of the week I seemed to be coming down with a sore throat and a cold. I continued to be ill that weekend, and didn't get better.

What It Was Like to be Ill

I am aware that in making a list of everything I have done in the years since becoming ill with ME, I might be giving the impression that I really wasn't very sick or perhaps, not sick at all. I was, and remain sick and I ascribe my ability to do all that I have done to a ruthless commitment to conserve my physical energy. I stuck to this whether or not it involved behaving in ways that looked strange, or were embarrassing to others or involved making what might have seemed unreasonable demands. Behaving in this way wasn't easy. There were many occasions when I was frustrated to the point of tears by having to ask for help – if there was anyone around to ask – for an apparently simple task (like unscrewing the lid to the petrol tank and holding the hose to put the petrol in). If I was somehow trapped in a situation where over-exertion was unavoidable, it could result in being bedridden for days afterwards. I was dependent on the kindness of both those closest to me and of perfect strangers. I was fortunate that when kindness had to be rewarded with payment, I was earning enough to afford it. That is not to say that I didn't experience exploitation and unkindness, as well.

That first weekend, and the following week, I was completely baffled and frustrated by my situation. I didn't have any of the normal symptoms of flu or of a cold, I just felt as if my body had ground to a halt. I was limp and exhausted in a way that would have made sense if I had just pushed myself to my last bit of energy climbing up a mountain or carrying a heavy load. It was quite strange to be that tired but not out of breath. If I tried to do anything, I started feeling dreadful – as you would if you were forced beyond exhaustion – and then my muscles just wouldn't do any more. In that state, the natural choice (and the only choice) is to go on lying down, but you assume that when you are tired and rest, you will stop being tired after a while. Except that 'after a while' never seems to arrive. Never having heard of ME, or of any illness that resembled this, I was in a state of confusion and disbelief. It is surreal: every moment you think 'this can't be happening, I'll wake up one morning and it will be fine'. If someone had said to me 'I don't believe in this illness' I would have replied 'I don't believe in it either!' Unfortunately, not believing in it didn't make any difference and this time it just went on and on.

The proponents of the psycho-social view of ME think that <u>believing in it</u> is what's <u>causing</u> it. In fact, <u>this</u> is the 'false illness belief' which must be challenged. The sooner we recognise that we have ME, the sooner we can respond by reorganising our lives to conserve every bit of <u>unnecessary</u> physical and mental exertion, <u>in order to create the possibility of recovery</u>, and in the hope that by doing so immediately, we will increase our chances of ultimately being able to return to a semblance of normal living, including returning to our jobs.

So this is where my saga begins to differ from that of those courageous, determined people who are convinced that the thing to do is to fight your illness. Many stories of people with ME recount struggles to keep going. They describe how people pushed themselves to go beyond the limits of what felt possible (but often they do not get very far, because the muscles do just shut down.) Predictably, and tragically, these brave and determined souls are the ones most likely to end up among the 25% who are severely and permanently disabled. Almost every piece of research, every description of ME along with every set of guidelines will include the observation that physical (and mental) exertion makes the symptoms worse, and may contribute to more serious and long-term disability. (Yet Graded Exercise Therapy is recommended as a treatment!) I remember the level of fear, amounting to terror, that I felt at the idea that someone – a psychiatrist, perhaps – might come along and say it was all in my head, and force me to run up and down the garden, not that I would have been able to. But I felt in my body what the consequences would be – a downward spiral of not being able to do it, collapsing in tears, having someone say this proved it was all emotional and I was just being silly and stubborn, and being driven on, to the point of......well, what? In fact, this scenario is one that is imposed on many people with ME (sometimes resulting in suicide, and sometimes in death [12] [13]) and probably is the fundamental reason why I am writing this book. I was lucky. It didn't happen to me. It shouldn't happen to anyone.

Despite being very busy and very active, and quite ambitious, and dedicated to the profession of psychotherapy, and helping people in a broader sense, I am very unwilling to be even slightly physically uncomfortable, and perhaps am also fundamentally lazy. I knew that muscular exertion would make me feel terrible, so my response was to figure out every possible way to conserve muscular exertion, and organise my life on that basis. This approach was reinforced by the leaflet from the ME Association, which said that the prognosis depended upon how much rest one was able to take during the first six months of the illness. It also stated that if you had been ill for two years, there was a 50% probability that you could be fully recovered by six years. So not any time soon!

I believe that this determined but selective initial 'laziness' is one of the main reasons that I was able to do so many things while ill, and have followed a (somewhat erratic!) trajectory of gradual recovery.

However I have always thought that resting was the most boring thing in the world, so I sought as many ways as possible to keep things interesting, within the extreme limits on both physical and mental activity imposed by the illness. The alternative would have been a constant state of angry frustration/despair – not particularly helpful towards recovery! In the early stages, I wrote a poem about the daffodils, which that April had experienced an unseasonable snowfall. The daffodils seemed able to be very still, quite contented to just be there and be daffodils, even in the adverse circumstances of being covered with snow! A good role model for an energetic person forced into stillness.

When it got warmer, and I was spending time lying in the garden, it occurred to me that if I studied everything that went on in one cubic inch of grass-covered earth, it could virtually fill a lifetime - the earth itself, its physical properties, and its geological history. The grass, what goes on in a blade of grass? Physiologically, chemically, how does it grow, how does photosynthesis work? And we haven't even got to the bacteria yet, let alone the ants and beetles. That seemed a useful metaphor for a life that was absolutely narrowed and restricted, yet still full of interesting things.

There were practical adjustments. Always an enthusiastic swimmer, my training in swimming and life-saving had taught me that our heads are very heavy – an important technique for survival in water for several hours depends on letting your head rest in the water except for taking the occasional quick couple of breaths. Trying to keep your head up out of the water will exhaust you after a short time. Applying this to ME, I learned to make sure to be in furniture (high-backed chairs or settees) and in physical positions in which my head was supported. When I returned to work, I could keep track of what was going on in a meeting only if my head was supported. If that wasn't possible, the physical effort of holding my head up, even when leaning on my elbows, would soon blot out any ability to understand what was going on. So I backed my chair up against walls, or draped myself over two chairs, if their backs were low, or leaned my head against one of the handles of my wheelchair. It is only in recent years that I have lost the habit of checking out any new place I go into, a pub or restaurant, for high-backed chairs or a place where I could lean against a wall. This one strategy for conserving energy seems to me one of the most effective, and essential. We wouldn't stand (or sit) holding up a ball that weighed 8 pounds for no particular reason, and we would expect to find it tiring. But, because in normal life we don't notice the effort constantly exerted in our neck and back muscles in order to hold up our heads, it isn't easy to appreciate how much difference to our well-being it can make if we just make keeping our heads supported a priority.

Taking this a step further, in the garden I noticed how easy it was to sit up or lie down in one of those light-weight, full-length canvas recliners. A slight lift of the arms and you can lean back as far as you like, as the back goes down and the part supporting your legs comes up. Another slight movement and you can be still resting, but sitting up enough to read, eat, or carry on a conversation. Or you can sit all the way up, to watch television, or type on a keyboard in your lap.

In the Park Avenue house, the rooms were big enough so that I could fit a recliner into each of the downstairs rooms. There is a big psychological difference between lying down on a settee and sitting up in a chair, let alone the difference between resting in a bedroom on your own or being downstairs as part of the life of your household. As your condition follows its unpredictable pattern, the recliner means having instant, easy access to complete rest when needed. Having to lie down for a few moments, or minutes, or hours, can be interspersed with normal activities, almost imperceptibly, without experiencing yourself, or being perceived by others, as an invalid who is 'having to lie down'.

When I got back to work, I was able to persuade the Department to allow me an executive-type chair, which both swivelled easily and allowed one to lean back into a relaxed position. It is provisions such as this which can facilitate a person with ME managing a job successfully. The difficulties for me, after an office move to an older building, included a very heavy front door, having an office on the first floor (no lift!), at the furthest point from the stairs, and the fact that the typing pool was at the furthest point from the stairs on the ground floor. Effectively, this meant that it was not possible for me to use their services. By the time I had walked the distance to the typing pool, I was too tired to figure out what I was supposed to be doing, let alone having to stand while explaining or proofreading and then go all the way back up. And down again, when the revised copy was ready. (Of course now we would all be doing our own typing on our PC's. Thanks to the loan of a PC by the then Finance Officer, Tony Murphy, I was one of the first to take up this trend.)

When I was first ill, I was too tired to sit up and type, or to write things out by hand, which made it impossible to do any office work or any personal correspondence with my far-flung family. This situation prevailed until my mother made me a gift of a dictating machine, and my daughter's then partner, Nick Hogg, gave up time to transcribe my letters and help with other administrative chores. Later, and with considerable difficulty, lying down with the keyboard on my lap and the monitor beside the settee, I learned to write in Wordstar. As I had been a technical typist for years mastering the keyboard was easy – the hard part was learning the differences between a typewriter and a PC. With our contemporary familiarity with technology, it may be difficult to imagine the challenge this presented for a woman of fifty, who was also very ill. The fact that I did successfully make the transition from a typewriter to a PC is one measure of my desperation not to let illness cut me off from the life I was used to living.

Going through my daily activities, there were many other short-cuts which I think most people with ME work out for themselves. One of the logistical dilemmas posed by the house where I lived was the fact that the downstairs loo was a relatively long walk down a passageway beyond the kitchen, and the upstairs loo was upstairs! My choices were to stay in bed and be isolated, but very near a loo, or go downstairs and have to wait as long as possible to minimise my exhausting walks through the kitchen and down the corridor – not easy when one of the symptoms of ME is a frequent need to urinate.

When kitchen tasks were unavoidable, I opted to bring water to a kettle in a light plastic jug rather than carrying a heavy kettle to the sink and filling it. I exchanged heavy frying pans for light-weight ones and I swapped heavier crockery for pretty plastic picnic plates. Necessary tasks had to be broken down into stages with rests in between, or done over a period of several days. Doors or drawers that were difficult to open had to be sorted out to make it easy. Ironing, when it was possible at all, could be done sitting on a high stool rather than standing. Better yet, I tried to have clothes that didn't need ironing. The need to minimise any 'long' walks or avoid going upstairs required constant advance planning. For example, it involved listing and collecting together everything I might need for the day before coming downstairs in the morning. (Not easy, when your brain, as well as your muscles, isn't working very well!)

And yet, despite all of these efforts to manage my condition I do not think my recovery would have been possible had I continued to live in such a big house. Fortunately, my circumstances permitted me to move to a very small flat for several months, where the bed, the bathroom, and the little kitchenette were illegally close together, and everything could be done within a few feet. It was during this time that I was doing the job as Principal Officer Health and one of the friends who drove me and provided wheel-chair assistance

(Juan Vizoso) also lived in a flat in the same house which meant that I was virtually chauffeured from door to door. The list of 'Things I Did While I Was Ill' was only made possible because they existed alongside a very long list of 'Things I Didn't Do', whilst shamelessly living like an invalid, being helped at every step of the way.

Recalling the early years when I was ill, there are a few memories I have of specific events that highlighted the symptoms of ME.

Mental Fatigue

In the very early months, I had not yet realised that mental effort would have an effect similar to physical exertion. In the quest for something to alleviate the endless boredom, I invited a friend who was working in the field of artificial intelligence to come round and talk to me about it. I had thought it sounded interesting, and an aspect of the modern world that one should know about.

Despite the fact that I was lying on the settee throughout, after an hour or so I was exhausted to the point of tears, unable to understand simple words, let alone any more complicated concepts. This was ample confirmation that mental exertion would have the same exhausting effect as physical effort.

Emotional Lability

Another feature of ME is emotional lability and this is used as part of the argument that ME is a psychiatric condition (soon to be included in DSM-5 in the newly invented category 'somatoform disorders').

One experience of this occurred when my daughter and her partner were out very late, and there was a knock at the door in the early hours of the morning. It was only a matter of a few seconds until the door was opened and they came in, having forgotten their keys. In that few seconds, there had been the predictable flash of 'is it the police with bad news?' which was dispelled almost immediately. However, I was sitting on the floor sobbing, for the next several minutes. Obviously, I wasn't sad, they were fine. It seemed to be a delayed and exaggerated response to that few seconds of intense emotion, and to be similar to the kind of emotional over-reaction that one would experience if extremely physically exhausted.

Another example of this happened sometime after I was in my new job, Principal Officer Health for Grimsby and Scunthorpe. I had spent a day on one of those group training exercises for higher levels of management, held in a suitably luxurious hotel. It was the kind of day I thoroughly enjoyed, having been a fan of group training for years. Also, being included in this particular event was a mark of my career success. This long but exhilarating day concluded with an excellent dinner, and much conviviality.

However, at the point where we were disbanding, I suddenly realised that I didn't have a hope of being able to make it to my car, which I had left in a nearby car park. Fortunately, I was able to catch the eye of the Finance Officer, and, with some embarrassment, I asked him if he would mind driving me to my car, even though it was right around the corner. As we set off, he was utterly baffled when, sobbing profusely, I explained between sobs that I was really happy, I had had a brilliant day, and it was just that I was very tired. (He was sufficiently alarmed by this to insist on driving me home, with a promise to help me collect my car the next day.) Here again, my sobbing was not in the least about being emotionally upset, it was entirely a response to the physical exhaustion of what had been a very enjoyable and rewarding day.

Post-Exertional Malaise

The term 'post-exertional malaise' is another frequently used term to describe the set of very unpleasant physical sensations which can follow exertion for a person with ME. Ramsay himself refers to delayed and prolonged fatigue following exercise. Although it is a somewhat controversial term, as most people would not use it in ordinary speech and it cannot be quantified by external observation, I think it is a distinct phenomenon, one that is qualitatively different from tiredness, emotional distress, or physical pain.

During the first months of my illness, before I had gone back to work, following the unfortunate venture into artificial intelligence, I made another ill-advised attempt to find a relatively harmless activity to fill in the long, boring days. This was to attend a one-day poetry workshop. I used to write quite a bit of rather mediocre poetry, and had enjoyed such workshops in the past.

The venue was a former primary school and it was equipped with the typically Spartan facilities that are generally provided for adult education and learning workshops. We were expected to sit around on the floor for quite a bit of it, and I remember the problems of remaining unsupported in a semi-sitting position for several hours. I more or less managed it during the day, but I made the mistake of returning for an evening event after a meal and a rest at home. Later that night, when I had gone to bed, I felt dreadful and I can only describe this feeling as one of an all-over, obscure but extreme unpleasantness which convinced me that I was quite likely to die during the night. A part of me was saying 'don't be silly, what would you be dying of' but I was mentally composing loving notes to the family, just in case. I wasn't frightened or upset, just feeling so physically bad that impending death seemed a rational prediction. I didn't die and over the next few days, I gradually reverted to my usual level of illness, but I didn't plan to go to any more poetry workshops for a while.

'Malaise' (literally, 'ill ease') is not a strong enough term to describe this feeling. Without involving actual physical pain, the sensation was certainly unpleasant enough to account for people with ME being quite frightened of a level of overexertion which might bring it on. And one can understand why people might have strong emotional responses to the prospect of being pushed to undergo Graded Exercise Therapy. But of course, these responses in themselves can be, and indeed are used, as further proof that we are psychiatrically disturbed.

This feeling of an overall dreadfulness is probably the result of inadequate delivery of oxygen to all of our tissues, caused at least to some extent by the stiffening of our red blood cells. Dr. Paul Cheney's report of the very low volume of blood flow in patients with ME is of interest here. (Dr. Cheney's work, along with a number of other studies of heart problems in CFS/ME can be found on the website of the ME Society of America, http://www.cfids-cab.org/MESA Cardiac Insufficiency Hypothesis [14]) I believe that the observations reported in these studies can be at least partially explained by Dr. Simpson's research on stiffened red blood cell populations. According to Dr. Simpson, aerobic exercise improves blood viscosity by making the cells more flexible, but anaerobic exercise produces a population change to a majority of the less flexible cells, this seems to me to confirm my personal theory that for people with ME, any exercise above a bare minimum becomes anaerobic.

'Psychiatric'?

At the time I became ill, I had been running a day centre for people with mental health problems for four years. During that time, the work that we were doing had gained a great deal of respect from the local psychiatrists. Our approach was based on my extensive reading and study in the field of psychology and psychotherapy, my experience of personal counselling and therapy, and more than ten years of previous experience in working with people who were labelled as 'mentally ill'.

For nine years, I had practiced group, individual and family therapy at Pashby House under the supervision of Dr. J.A. Ardis. I was very familiar with psychopharmacology as well as the newer approaches to psychotherapy including transactional analysis, non-directive (person-centred) therapy, the systems approach to working with families, and behaviourist approaches. This was in addition to extensive study of the theory and practice of community therapy

With this background, knowledge and experience, I felt very well-equipped to question my first doctor's judgement that my ME 'must be psychiatric'. I was very aware of the fact that I had nothing to feel unusually sad, guilty or anxious about. The worst thing about my life was that there was too much of it! I knew what my 'issues' were and had been, and I had willingly spent hours of therapy and training dealing with them. Had my ME been something that was amenable to resolution through psychotherapy, sorting it out would have been pretty straightforward! But the incapacity that I experienced was definitely physical, and it was very frightening. However, once I knew that there was no test for it, and no treatment other than rest, I saw no point whatever in troubling a doctor further and after the encounters described earlier, I didn't.

What I undoubtedly did have was an extreme fear of having it diagnosed as psychological and being forced to exercise. In fact, you could say that the main feature of my contribution to this book is an attempt on my part to counteract the cultural trends and the recommendations which would label us as having a psychiatric problem and needing to be motivated and coerced into exercise to an extent that can make us more disabled, for longer, or can even – as has only recently been acknowledged – result in death. [15]

These harmful consequences of enforced exercise have been recognised, for example by Twisk and Maes : "So, it can be concluded that the efficacy claim for CBT/GET is false. But what is more important, is the fact that numerous studies support the thesis that exertion, and thus GET, can physically harm the majority of the ME/CFS patients." [16]

My criticisms of the group of psychiatrists who are working hard to get ME labelled as a psychiatric complaint, and have it listed alongside hypochondria, malingering, and psychosomatic illnesses – illnesses which are believed to have been brought about by the stress responses of an anxious personality – are based on, among other things, the lack of respect which they show to their own profession.

When reading their research papers and their justifications for their beliefs, one can sense a rather desperate search for something which would justify this labelling. People who have ME do not have any greater incidence of depression or anxiety than is present in the general population. If the subjects of a particular piece of research have been designated as having ME (or CFS) from a diagnostic list which <u>requires</u> 'post-exertional malaise' as a symptom, people who have depression will be eliminated because, in their case, exercise improves the mood. If, however, post-exertional malaise is <u>included but not required</u> (as in the Oxford guidelines), the population chosen will include ME sufferers but is also very likely to include a number of people who are suffering from depression, and not from ME. In this case, the research results would not prove anything about ME. And if the symptom 'post- exertional malaise' is used to <u>exclude</u> people from the patient group being researched (some people believe this may have applied to subjects chosen for the PACE Trial) then **no one who has ME will be included in that group, and any report of research results which did not indicate clearly that the research was not relevant to people with ME would have to be regarded as unethical.**

(For further discussion of these issues, see the review of Manu's book, 'The Psychopathology of Functional Somatic Syndromes' by Anthony Komaroff [17]. See also the conclusion in S. Song and L.A. Jason [18] noting that 'chronic fatigue secondary to psychiatric conditions' is distinct from CFS. Maes and Twisk [19] refer to an article stating that "ME/CFS can be differentiated with 100% accuracy from depression." [20] As noted earlier, their research reports [16] also say unequivocally that CBT and GET can be harmful for people with ME/CFS.

People who have ME may also, very realistically, be frightened and upset at finding themselves so disabled, without any visible reason or explanation. It is notable that the history of many, if not most people who become ill with ME has a striking absence of the kind of narrative that would lead to a serious psychiatric problem. I would expect any responsible psychotherapist to consider what kind of traumatic history would have to be the precursor to the sudden inception of such severe and multiple disabling symptoms. If there is no credible answer to that question within the client's narrative, a therapist's professional integrity would require a referral on for physical investigation. As the psychiatrists mentioned in the first part of Dr. Simpson's account (p. 13) were reported as saying, the honest psychiatric response has to be 'I do not know what this person is suffering from, but it does not fall within my field.'

The level of disability, together with its dire consequences (strain on relationships, loss of employment and income) is realistically very upsetting and demoralising. It is not neurotic to be upset by such events. But this level of distress, along with the emotional lability which is a symptom of the illness, can be wilfully misinterpreted as the further manifestations of a neurotic personality.

It is not necessary, I hope, to spell out the appropriate response to any psychiatrist or psychotherapist who appeared to be insisting that a client with a physical illness, and without a history that could offer a psychiatric explanation, was suffering from a psychiatric complaint, simply in order to make money out of treating them. It appears to me ironic that a psychiatrist whose own career is dependent on promoting the psychiatric model of ME has been alleged to have referred to people with ME as 'the least deserving of the sick', and 'scenting the possibility of a career'. [9] Most people who become ill with ME have had careers considerably more lucrative than that available through medical insurance or Incapacity Benefit. In the history of any person with ME, I do not believe that you could find an event or chain of events so traumatic as to produce, overnight, such a major set of physical limitations. It is interesting to read in Komaroff's review of the book by Manu (full reference given above) that when the author began to write the book he was convinced that ME was a psychosocial disorder, and by the time he had finished it, he was sure that it wasn't. It seems that he was persuaded by the information he gained in the course of his research.

Critics of my views can certainly point to me as an example of a neurotic personality with a history of going to counsellors and psychotherapists. They can hardly point to me as a person who would have rejected psychiatric help for a psychiatric problem!

I believe that 'being professional' requires us to behave with courtesy and respect toward the individuals who come to us for our professional services.

I believe that individuals who come to us with medical or psychiatric problems have a right to careful and thorough diagnostic procedures, appropriate referral, and to treatments which will help, not harm them.

And I am passionately concerned about the plight of people who have ME and are treated without respect, without proper professional courtesy and care, and offered so-called 'treatments' which will make them worse. We are the least able to fight our own battles, and most in need of help in doing so. I hope that this book will prove a useful tool in this cause.

(A wry postscript to the above is that the view that ME is the choice of hypochondriacs and malingerers is quite insulting to those two groups: no hypochondriac with a grain of sense would choose to complain of such a far-fetched collection of symptoms; and no malingerer worth his salt would stay with ME once he found out the level of insult and abuse which this illness attracts – he would immediately change his choice to an illness that might generate a bit more sympathy!)

My Story continues after the next Chapter...

Most ME people exhibit an unquenchable thirst for information about ME. Unfortunately this demand has been met by the publication of books which have the potential to mislead the reader. As a result, many ME people hold strong views based upon what they have read. The objective of this section is to provide some insight into what has been published in books on ME, when assessed from the viewpoint of Ramsay's concepts. The books are a random selection from the library of the Dunedin ME Information and Support Service and they convey such a diversity of opinions it was considered that such a review was necessary.

Books Written by Non-Physicians

1. Jeffreys T. The mile-high staircase. Hodder and Stoughton, Auckland, 1982.

Summary. This book should be compulsory reading for all carers and relatives of people with ME. The quality of the writing reflects the academic background of the author, who describes with clarity and vigour the devastating aftermath of developing an unknown and not understood illness in 1977. She describes graphically her slow improvement in well-being and the rapid return of her symptoms during a rollercoaster existence of severe illness and semi-wellness, and the chance events which after three years led her to recognise that she had ME.

Dr Jeffreys has a PhD in English Literature and Social History and was holding a research-orientated appointment. The onset of her illness was gradual, beginning with abdominal pains, followed eventually by increasing weakness which became obvious when climbing the stairs to her home. She wrote, *"Gradually I discovered something new about the world. It was an uphill world. Everywhere there were stairs, stairs, stairs. They leered at me, mocked me."*

Despite the gradual spread of a body wide pain, all tests ordered by physicians were negative and she gave up working. Neither the attention of a helpful physician nor a hospital admission provided relief. The writer exhibits signs of a degree of antipathy towards the medical profession, which was not relieved by the failure to recognise the nature of her illness. She wrote, *"Are most doctors too busy for ordinary politeness, or is it not considered necessary with an ill person? The politeness doesn't cost much, and possibly it helps the patient to get better faster."* So it is interesting that in Professor Natelson's book on fatigue he included a chapter titled "Understanding the doctor," which provides some frank insights into doctor training. He wrote, "*Unfortunately, the youth and relative inexperience of most medical students makes them highly susceptible to the peer pressure that changes a considerate young doctor-to-be into someone who can be described by the 3 Bs – brash, boorish and bullying – in addition to being unkind and a poor listener.*" This would tend to confirm Dr. Jeffrey's insights.

As the severity of her illness progressed, she describes graphically the nature of her pains and the level of her weakness, and at some points, what she refers to as levels of madness, and at times she contemplated suicide. As a hospital patient she was not impressed by the treatment of other patients, so it is not surprising that she wrote, "*Most of all, I hated the solemnity of hospital life. When people in white coats came, I wanted to say something funny,*" and,

> *The general solemnity of the medical profession is supposed to convey authority, responsibility, respectability and omniscience, if not omnipotence. This is all part of the healing process. The patient looks up to the doctor. He is super-self-confident, which tells the patient she is in good hands. This gives her the confidence to get better. But does it? I was dazed and confused. What I longed for, for weeks and months was a two- minute chat.*

Matters came to a head when she was told she was to have an X-ray, and she wanted to know why this was necessary, but no explanation was forthcoming. Eventually a professor arrived to tell her that either she had the X-ray or she might as well check out of hospital. She opted to check out, but learned later that as many of her symptoms occurred also with cancer, that was the reason for the X-ray. But no one had explained this to her.

At home, she was bolstered by visits from friends, but seven months after the onset she was still very unwell, despite a regimen of vitamin and mineral supplements, with raw vegetables, fruits, nuts and fish. Acupuncture was not helpful. After several months of illness she visited a naturopath who told her she had some sort of adrenal crisis and would take two years to get over it!

A second hospitalisation, in a different hospital, in a private room was a different experience, even though all the extensive laboratory tests were negative. But after several weeks she realised that she was feeling better, although an identified muscle weakness led to the provision of an exercise regime by a physiotherapist.

After discharge from hospital, she overdid her physical resources during her first day shopping and relapsed and experienced another six months of illness. She noted that for the first two or three weeks she would be severely unwell, with poor nights and depression. Then there would be a slow reduction in symptom severity and by the fifth week, brief periods of walking were possible. She noted that during this episode she tried every "alternative" health measure she could find. However she did learn that rest was imperative and activity was fatal!

Two months later after she had been able to walk around the house, because she felt so well, another visit to see a film – with stairs to climb, led to another relapse and a few more weeks in bed. In April 1978 she returned to New Zealand and was admitted to hospital the following month. After some weeks she discovered the joys of a physiotherapy pool, where the buoyancy allowed her to exercise without effort. But on her second session, she swam a little, had overdone it and next morning was too weak to go to the pool.

Eventually she was given a diagnosis of psychosomatic illness. The confirmation of the diagnosis rekindled thoughts of suicide, which were rejected when she realised that this would simply confirm the idea of a neurotic woman. She continued to enjoy the benefits of the heated pool and three months later was walking a mile a day. A New Zealand naturopath also claimed the problem was her adrenals. At the end of July she returned to Sydney, but without her carer and returned to work.

When the prospect of a group trip to China arose, she sought medical advice, and she was told there was no reason why she should not make the trip. Among the various things which had to be done were some immunizations. Even though the injections were spaced a week apart, after the anti-typhoid injection, "...*things started going wrong.*" After a night of high and low temperature, there was a relentless decline in wellbeing, which would persist for another five months. She was correct on blaming the immunization, which I have found changes the shape populations of red blood cells.

When her carer came to Sydney, he brought with him some information about the Royal Free Disease. Despite early difficulties in a search for information about the disease, a friend located a copy of the Nursing Times with most of the issue devoted to Royal Free Disease. Subsequently, they were able to tape a discussion by an English doctor who was a sufferer. All this was the follow up to a symposium on the topic which had been held in England in April. Even though the disorder had been recognised since the 1930s, it was neglected and unknown. She wrote *"Why? One purpose of this book is an attempt to answer that question, to show something of the background against which such a terrible oversight could occur."* She wrote also

> *Of course, it must be hard to get interested in an illness which doesn't kill, disfigure or deform, which hasn't got the courtesy to announce its presence with a dramatic abnormality in the blood, the spinal fluid, the nerves, muscles or faeces, a disease which tends to make sufferers difficult people to be with, incapable of normal activity.*

But now she knew that there is an abnormality of the blood which does not show up in usual blood tests.

Dr. Jeffreys was quite correct in stating, "M.E. is one of the 'poor relations' in a hierarchy of diseases. By that I mean a hierarchy of priorities, a hierarchy based on how much money, brains, and energy is available to tackle a medical problem." Only recently in the UK has the problem of ME generated political interest. Further investigations by helpful friends led to the arrival of three articles on ME all of which allowed her to confirm her self-diagnosis, but she and her carer recognised the need to have a medical certificate which confirmed the diagnosis. And eventually she achieved that goal.

Then they returned to New Zealand "....frail, sick and in a wheelchair" She noted that this time the illness was different "...I was jumpy, restless and had difficulty concentrating. It was most peculiar. I was weak and moved slowly, and yet at the same time I couldn't relax, I couldn't settle in one place. I could neither read nor do any writing." As a result she recognised that she needed medical help, which lead to a doctor's prescription for three drugs. She took one third of the recommended dose and slept for almost 24 hours – but woke into a different world. She felt, "relaxed, happy and optimistic." Then she met another woman with an undiagnosed illness of five years duration, and compared medical histories. The similarities suggested she might have ME.

After a celebration of the purchase of a new house, a head cold preceded another relapse, despite resting for three days. A problem arose from the effects of the relapse on the family. How was it possible to be well for three months and then become sick again? It seemed that they did not believe the story of the strange disease. In her search for relief, she tried steroids which had been recommended, but they made her symptoms worse.

After two months of sickness she moved into her new house, and the move required that she search for a new GP. The selected doctor was sympathetic – and ordered blood tests which showed that there were abnormal (but not understood) values for immune globulins. So in September 1979, after two years of illness, she was finally "allowed" to be ill. When she suggested to her friend with ME? that she should have the same test done she followed the advice and had the same result.

When trying to understand what had caused the disease, she concluded that what was missing from the medical literature was some input from the patients. She wrote

> *It is this literature which shapes the thinking of generations of doctors. Why is not a patient's account included in medical writings? Even if all that the patient can say is 'P.S. It's bloody awful.' It is the missing ingredient. If it isn't there, the reader sees the disease as a detached entity, a label fastened onto a human being and it is the label which comes alive, not the patient. There are no words. No vocabulary of illness. We experience it. We endure it. And afterwards, if we're lucky and recover, we forget it.*

Later there is a vigorous examination of psychosomatic illness as a diagnosis. She summarised and graded the effectiveness of the various physicians she had been involved with and only 3 of 12 scored an A while 4 were graded D. However, in view of my findings concerning the importance of blood flow, it needs to be recognised that the physicians were faced with a problem involving blood rheology, a science they had never been taught about.

In her discerning fashion, Dr. Jeffreys has provided a record of her experience of the ups and downs in ME, which are sure to strike a chord with any who have the problem – whether recognised or not. Even though it is 25 years since publication, her description of ME is just as valid today as it was then.

Even though I have never met Dr. Jeffreys I can recall her reclining on a couch at the rear of the lecture hall, during the Cambridge Symposium.

2. Wilkinson S. M.E. and you: A survivor's guide to post-viral syndrome. Thorsons Publishers Limited, Wellingborough, 1988.

Summary. The author's choice of post-viral syndrome is a good reason for not recommending this book as background reading for any ME sufferer. At the time of writing (1988) a general lack of information and doctor's attitudes would be good reasons for ME sufferers to explore alternative and/or complementary services to seek an understanding of their health problems. Even though a small number of ME people consider that they benefited from one or more of the costly treatments available, it needs to be emphasised that there is no scientific support for the efficacy of "natural" therapies.

From the viewpoint of Ramsay's Disease, it is unfortunate that the author should equate ME with post-viral syndrome (PVS). As this is an account of the author's experience of his illness, he includes the problems of finding a sympathetic doctor, and he notes his "incredible" relief on eventually gaining a diagnosis. In marked contrast to Toni Jeffreys' experience he wrote (p13)

> *With renewed strength I returned to my therapies. I was determined to get the virus out of my system, or at least to learn how to keep it well and truly under control. My confidence in the therapies was well founded. For months now I have been free of all of the major symptoms, for the first time since the illness started. When I think back to how ill I was, this seems an unbelievable achievement, but even now, every day brings another small improvement. There are still relapses, times of weakness and tiredness, but these can be controlled and they pass quickly.*

He wrote also:

> *Living with ME is a constant exercise in the fine art of self-awareness. Gradually you learn about your own tolerances and limitations; how much you can do without suffering for it later; how long you can concentrate; how late you can stay up; how early you can rise; how much you can work or play or write or talk or watch TV, or drink, or think or listen or walk or read or eat or...or...or. All of these things which you used to take for granted, suddenly have to be measured and carefully considered. You have to remain constantly aware of your resources of strength and to take good care that you do not exhaust them." (p16)*

However, this very good advice was tempered by the following statement. "*Of course your limitations will be completely different from anyone else's.*" However, in my experience, an ME sufferer would need to be well on the way to recovery before he or she was able to consider their limitations.

The author expressed the very definite opinion that, "Myalgic encephalomyelitis is caused by a virus – probably one of the 80 or more viruses known as the "entero" virus group, which enter the body through the digestive system and which affect the brain, nerves and muscles of the sufferer." But the failure to recognise that some ME cases have non-viral causes, is an indication that his concept is on shaky foundations.

In different places in the text, he notes the symptoms of ME, viz. extreme tiredness, fatigue, coldness, muscular pain and swelling, back and head pain, memory lapses, lack of comprehension and rapid mood swings. Although he referred to a patient in remission, who relapsed, there was no comment about how remissions could occur during a persistent viral infection. Even though he recognised that a minority will suffer from the illness for years, he stated, "*The illness continues for a period of weeks or months (often not more than eight months) then the patient starts to improve. Day by day the symptoms recede and the patient begins to feel human again."* However, in introducing concepts such as "energy levels" and a need to "listen" to your emotions to explain the nature of ME, the author moves into concepts of dubious value.

Although he commented on the implications of about 20 symptoms it is unclear that he had a clear understanding of the physiology of the changes he discussed. But it is of importance that he should recognise "tiredness" as the most significant symptom.

Much has been written about the role of Candida in ME. A colleague (Dr. Brett Shand) searched for anti-Candida antibodies in ME people and in randomly selected hospital patients. His results showed that Candida antibodies were much more frequent in hospital patients than in ME people.

In a chapter on treatment, the author favoured alternative medicine and noted,

> *Alternative therapies spring from an entirely different understanding of health from orthodox medicine. Traditional medical practitioners tend to think of the body as a machine, and they will treat the parts of the machine that are not working smoothly. In this sense they treat the disease and not the patient. Alternative practitioners are more likely to think of the patient as a whole unit (hence the term 'holistic medicine') composed of mind and body: they believe that both these aspects of self must be treated to cure any problem.*

This simplistic concept of medicine in general, and the role of alternative practitioners tends to draw attention to the importance of the lack of an agreed pathophysiology for ME which would provide a basis for treatment.

Given that the concepts of orthodox vs. alternative medicine are controversial, it is not surprising that his list of therapies is equally controversial. He discussed acupuncture, acupressure, aromatherapy, autogenic training, Bach flower remedies, colonic irrigation, exercise, healing, herbalism, homeopathy, hydrotherapy, hypnosis and auto-hypnosis, kinesiology, massage, meditation, reflexology, relaxation, royal jelly, tissue salts, vitamins and diet supplements and yoga. Quite apart from the costs of some of these treatments, a major difficulty in accepting that any might be helpful is the lack of assessment by placebo controlled, double-blinded studies.

However, his approach to exercise is acceptable and he noted, *"During convalescence, exercise becomes both necessary and beneficial,"* and he recommended starting, *"...to take a little exercise regularly."* Because he quoted no references it is unclear if the author was aware of those studies which showed that one of the effects of exercise was to reduce blood viscosity.

At the beginning of the chapter, the author stated that help was at hand, *"...if you find the right therapy."* I agree with this idea, and when I learn from a patient that they have received benefit from an unexpected quarter, I advise them to persist with the treatment. It is not important that there is no explanation for the perceived benefit. If a treatment provides an individual with benefit, then he/she should stick with it. But be prepared for the fact that the treatment may not help others.

In writing about the importance of maintaining a positive attitude, the author made claims which would be difficult to substantiate. For example, his conclusion

Developing the right attitude to your illness will reduce your suffering, make life easier for you and your carers and result in a quicker recovery. The wrong attitude will have exactly the reverse effect, and can undo much of the good done by any therapy you may try.

In other words, if a therapy does not work, the fault lies with the attitude of the sufferer. It is difficult to reconcile such a concept with the detailed history of events documented by Dr. Toni Jeffreys.

Dr Simpson is correct in suggesting that blaming the sufferer's attitude for failure to get better is both incorrect and unhelpful. But our culture insists that we must 'fight' illness and disability, and most ME sufferers share this attitude, and lived determinedly active and healthy lives until they became ill. ME is a counter-cultural illness: recovery requires that we do the opposite of 'fighting' – we have to learn to accept the limitations on activity which the illness imposes, if we are to have any chance of ultimate recovery. But to 'give in' without losing self-respect is an incredible challenge in our culture. People with ME need to learn, quickly, that physical rest is the correct form of 'fighting', and be courageous about insisting that others respect this.

As stated elsewhere, Dr. Simpson encourages patient-limited, slightly incremental gentle exercise in order to avoid the increased blood viscosity caused by complete inactivity. Gentle exercise improves blood viscosity, more strenuous exercise (which in the case of a person with ME, can mean any but the most limited) makes it worse. This is why he says that the patient must be in control – only the patient can know the limits of what he or she can do at a particular time. He agrees that rest is essential especially in the acute, early stage, and entirely disagrees with the idea that forcing exercise on people with ME could possibly be helpful.

A chapter titled, "For the carers," notes

Just as the sufferer must make adjustments to their physical lifestyle, so must the carer; you must allow more time for those extra chores, plan your time and energy wisely and decide what are priorities and what can wait. .....Tying yourself completely to the sufferer for 24 hours a day is the fastest way to wear yourself down, utterly destroying the strength and resilience that both of you need badly. Consciously plan ahead, to set aside fun time for yourself, to get away from all the limitations of ME.

Subsequently he wrote

Finally, the one thing the sufferer needs from people round about, more than anything else is optimism, the belief that in the not too distant future the sufferer will be back in ruddy health. Because ME is a long and serious illness, it is all too easy for the sufferer to lose their sense of direction, their aims and their goals.

Unfortunately, this sound advice may have relevance only when the sufferer has recovered sufficiently even to think about the future.

3. March C. (editor). Knowing ME. The Women's Press Limited, London 1998.

Summary. While there are many pockets of interest in some contributions, it is doubtful that the book provides the information needed to "Know ME," without some reference to the material which had been published up to the year of publication. For that reason it is difficult to reconcile the contents of the book with its title. While comments on the disabling nature of the disorder pervade the book, there is almost a total absence of references to medical assistance. Either the available information was unknown to the many contributors, or it was ignored. Therefore it seems reasonable to ask how ME can be known if the available information is not made use of. In my opinion this book will provide little useful information about ME.

In the introduction the editor wrote, "The title of the book, "Knowing ME," is intended to reflect the different ways in which women respond to this syndrome and the variety of knowledge gained by those who live with it." But her concept of ME is that it is equivalent to CFS, and it was noted, "Here the abbreviation that has been adopted is a simplified one, CFS, which stands for Chronic Fatigue Syndrome." There is no indication that she was aware of the controversy over nomenclature, and her idea was that ME is "…only one kind of chronic fatigue," ignoring the other health problems of those disabled by ME.

The 30 contributors provided viewpoints which ranged from one and a half to fifteen pages in length, with the majority comprising two to three pages. Although several contributors provided a lesbian perspective, their experience was not much different from that of black, brown or white women.

A surprising feature of virtually all contributors was the apparent rejection of the available information about ME. Maybe this was due to the lack of access to medical libraries, although ME Support Groups are good sources of information. Surprisingly, for an English publication, Ramsay's work was not mentioned, nor was the Cambridge Symposium on ME referred to.

In Part 1, "Diagnosis, definitions and decisions," 23 contributors filled 60 pages with their personal experiences and how ME changed their pattern of living. While some cases began in the late 1960s and early 1970s, many became ill in the early 1990s. In general, their experience reflected the experience of others, and there were major problems in obtaining a diagnosis, with frequent referrals to psychiatrists for psychosomatic disorders.

Antidepressants were offered frequently as a treatment for anxiety, and a lack of effective treatment by physicians led to the exploration of alternative medicine. Unfortunately, many accounts are un-dated making it impossible to determine what information about ME was available at that time.

Part 2, is titled, "Family, friends and community," and 57 pages were contributed by ten writers. A high school girl provided her experience of several years of suffering without a diagnosis, but it is not clear if medical help was sought after a school teacher suggested she was a classic case of ME. Gradually she returned to near-normal functioning. A writer who discussed ME and pregnancy, noted that, "…the majority of women find that their ME symptoms improve during pregnancy." Although there is general recognition that the beneficial effects noted during pregnancy relate to the 40% to 50% increase in blood volume, which increases progressively from about the eighth week of gestation, this was not noted. However, with the increase in volume, blood viscosity would be reduced and capillary blood flow would be improved. There was a discussion about whether or not women with ME should plan a pregnancy, and it was noted, *"Even the national ME organisation can only give general advice, without any definite answer."* In addition, medical advice was very variable. This was followed by comments concerning motherhood of lesbians with ME, and where advice could be obtained. A lesbian gave her account of eight years with ME, at a time when she had improved greatly. However, there was no mention of any medical involvement, although a shiatsu practitioner was mentioned.

Part 3, is a 63 page discussion by 18 contributors on the topic, "Healing ourselves." In one case where, *"...my GP offered me kindness and pep talks,"* alternative medical help was sought. This provided temporary improvement, but at high cost. After five years of sickness, she found a Chinese herbal medicine, and after four months treatment was much better but not fully recovered.

Another long-term case seems to have totally abandoned medical care. She uses self-help acupressure, Chinese food herbs and transcendental meditation. In addition she makes use of alternative healers and has an interest in spiritual matters.

A physiotherapist with ME found a sympathetic GP who believed in ME, but who referred her to a specialist who did not. Subsequently, she was referred to another consultant who believed in ME and sent her for aerobic exercises. She noted, *"Because someone has decided that aerobic exercise is good for ME and someone is doing a study to prove it. Not on me they're not."*

Another writer, presumably suffering from ME, with the support of a herbalist, believed that improvement would follow when approached at five different levels: namely the physical, the emotional, the psychological, the intellectual and the spiritual. These different levels were described under the following headings. Diet, massage/hugging, laughter, painting, exercise, relaxation, decoration and atmosphere, herbal medicine and spiritual healing. The writer noted,

> *The most valuable thing that I was able to do for myself was to adjust the inner image of myself and my illness. I have since learned that this is a technique commonly used in hypnosis; though I was not aware of it before, intuitively I felt that it would help me to recover.*

It is very difficult to relate this experience to that of others with ME, and could lead to doubts about whether or not ME was involved.

From a psychotherapeutic perspective, massage, hugging, and laughter could all have positive effects on the internal environment via the activity of neurotransmitters responsive to physical contact and laughter. Relaxation in ME is absolutely essential, and a pleasant environment would also contribute to overall well-being. Cultivating a creative outlet, providing it were one not involving much physical effort, could also be positive. Gentle exercise – but only if strictly controlled by the patient in order to stay within the limits set by the illness – could be helpful. As stated earlier, maintaining self-respect in the face of cultural attitudes to the 'giving in' essential to recovery from ME would be a particularly useful way to 'adjust to the inner image of myself and my illness'.

In marked contrast was the experience of a woman who had had ME for three and a half years who wrote, "I was plunged into the nightmare world of good days and bad days, relapses and remissions and the overwhelming sensation of being exhausted right to my inner core." Later she noted, "ME has brought terrifyingly unexpected relapses in health and at the same time wonderfully unexpected discoveries." She learned how great her parents were; she learned about friendship; she learned that her body needed to be looked after; she learned to be disciplined and to have an open mind. At no point did she mention medical services, and concluded, "ME has taken so much away from me, and yet through having it, I have learned so much that it has made my life richer."

Another woman in her third year with ME recorded that she had begun and eventually completed a two-year-long diploma course. She stated that she had pushed herself a lot, which made her ME worse. *"For me, the important thing was to recognise what was happening to me and to stop – no matter what."* There was no mention of treatments, but she was helped by the fact that both staff and course members were ME-friendly.

In contrast to most accounts was a contribution titled, "Fantasies, realities and a bit of common sense," which noted, "*…many people accept the holistic philosophy uncritically.*" But in writing, "*There is an ever-expanding junk literature of illness, which offers some extremely natty accounts of emotional or spiritual causes of illness,*" the author made it plain that such material was unhelpful, and she was very critical of the "illness personality." She drew attention to the fact that psychologists had the most to gain, "*…from simplistic ideas of illness personality.*" A discussion of "ME personality," began, "*Like other poorly understood illnesses, ME is surrounded by myths and fantasies. Religious and scientific experts both resort to magic to fill in the gaps in their knowledge.*" The author wrote, "*In Belinda Dawes and Damien Downing's (see later) experience, almost all people with ME are goal-oriented and '…strive hard to gain recognition and approval' because they suffer from a '…deep-seated lack of self-acceptance.'* "Later it was stated, "*What Dawes and Downing seem to ignore is that fighting illness rather than giving in to it, is the culturally acceptable form of behaviour.*" This is the only reference to a book by medically trained authors.

Another concept of the "ME personality" is that it is the avoidance of activity that leads to a chronic form of ME. "Apparently, some deluded people believe that they're ill, and therefore indulge in "illness behaviour". They stop going out and stay in bed, with the result that they get out of condition, and feel depressed." The writer concluded, "I use common sense to guide me when I wade through the ME literature, pore over statistics and weigh up benefits of various treatments and diets." Unfortunately, the writer had nothing to report about her findings when assessing the ME literature.

> People who get sick with ME have often been highly motivated, energetic, hard-working individuals, the type who ignore illness and 'just get on with it', as our culture increasingly pressures us to do. After they get sick, they are forced, by the nature of the illness, to minimise physical and mental exertion, or pay a severe price in worsening of symptoms and increasing their level of disability. Those determined to give ME a psychiatric label call this 'de-conditioning', 'exercise avoidance', and ascribe it – the whole illness – to 'illness beliefs'. The so-called 'illness beliefs' formed by people suffering from ME are based on fact – exertion beyond the limits imposed by the illness makes them worse. Suddenly acquiring a major disability for no obvious reason is an extremely distressing event, and being treated as though you are crazy, especially by those who have the power to force you to do things which will increase your pain and disability, is tantamount to torture, both emotional and physical. And I defy any psychiatrist to find a sound **psychiatric explanation** for the **sudden and complete change** which occurs when a person becomes ill with ME.

Another contributor with a four and a half year history of ME, discussing celibacy and ME, concluded, "Through having ME I have learned to appreciate the calmer things in life, and being lover-free has given me uncluttered time to be with myself, my thoughts and my feelings." She noted, "…sex and relationships have not been priorities."

The positive consequences which can follow from ME were set out by a black professional woman, whose career was cut short by ME. After a year of ME she wrote

> *Acknowledging and accepting the vast impact ME has had on my life, has consequently rendered the condition less important, and is enabling me to move forward slowly. For example, last summer I was consumed with anger, very frightened, struggling to keep depression at bay and in a lot of pain. I had difficulty in envisaging a future, and when I did it appeared bleak. In contrast, I am now excited by the future and view the coming summer as a brand-new beginning, a welcome gift waiting to be opened, and wherever it leads I will willingly follow. I have had to re-evaluate and reorganise my whole life.*

During recovery she did three hours a week of voluntary work and built new friendships. As a part of the healing process she welcomed, "*…the freedom to plan and define my days, and to give something back to society through voluntary work.*" She concluded, "*Now it also serves as a reminder of how much I still have to offer in spite of being afflicted by a chronic illness.*"

Part 4 is titled, "Benefits, rights and beyond." A two-page account reflected the problems of ME people, because they do not look unwell. In 1995, an Invalidity Benefit was denied because the medical officer considered that the applicant, "*…looked well and seemed cheerful and had been ill long enough.*" In appealing the decision, the applicant was denied permission to present pamphlets from the ME Association, which outlined how ME affected chronic cases. In essence, the 15 minute assessment by the medical officer was taken to outweigh the applicant's testimony, plus the written contributions from her GP, consultant and carer. A year later she had not learned of the appeal decision.

"ME and disability," is the title of an interesting discussion of different models of disability. While the medical model says that you are disabled by what is "wrong" with you, the social model concerns the way in which individuals, *"…are discriminated against or are excluded from participation in society."* Lack of wheelchair access to buildings was given as an example. It was noted *"Part of the impairment of ME is undoubtedly caused by the way it disables those of us who have it.* The writer concluded, *"This strengthens me against the isolation which is a key facet of life with ME. With this attitude, I remind myself that my exclusion is not an inevitable part of my illness, but a result of current social construction, and thus open to challenge."*

The concept of a "social model of disability," was discussed by another writer, who rarely left her flat because of her ME. She maintained a reluctance to use a wheelchair, because she thought that people in wheelchairs were completely dependent and helpless. But as soon as she was persuaded to use a wheelchair, her perception changed.

> *As soon as I got into the chair, I experienced the strongest feeling of liberation I have ever felt in my life. To move around is both pleasurable and empowering; if your mobility is restricted, that is deprivation. I still feel that liberation every time I use a wheelchair.*

In a general discussion of the social and medical models of disability, the writer stated

> *…the world is designed for able bodied people and takes little account of people with impairments. Because of this, people with various kinds of impairments are automatically excluded from many different places and activities. Such views led to disabled people arguing that their needs in areas such as transport, housing and education need to be addressed.*

However, because of her ME, the writer was unhappy with the social model of disability, and she was concerned about her image as a wheelchair user, when in some places she was ambulant. But she concluded

> *"In spite of my problem with the social model of disability, it has made a great difference to me. When I first became really ill with ME, I had many problems. I viewed them as the inevitable consequence of the illness and as the illness went on and on, I felt more and more hopeless. The social model of disability taught me that things which seem tragic and inevitable are not necessarily so."*

The final section of the book concerns outlines of the therapies for ME, offered by homeopathy, traditional Chinese medicine and herbalism. While each of the discussions was interesting and informative, if such treatments were effective, then why have they not been evaluated in controlled trials so that more people might be treated? An interesting aside is that, in the article on herbalism, Dr. Charles Shepherd's book, "Living with ME", is given as the reference for the use of evening primrose oil.

4. Franklin M, Sullivan J. M.E. What is it? Have you got it? How to get better, Century Hutchinson Limited, London, 1989.

Summary. This is an easy reading account of some of what has been written about ME, with some case histories and other useful information for ME people. However, there are no comments which would indicate that the authors really got to grips with the problem. While they favoured a viral cause, they did not attempt to explain how a virus could cause fatigue which may vary in intensity from hour to hour. Perhaps it should be read after the "Mile-high staircase."

Two journalists provide their interpretation of various aspects of ME, to some extent written around a small number of case histories. Unfortunately, only the first edition of Ramsay's book was available, so prominence was given to the post-viral syndrome. It could be of significance that there was an article in an English newspaper in June 1986 which stimulated a very large public response and drew attention to the medical attitude towards ME. It is worth noting with regard to that date that our report of poor filterability of ME blood was accepted in September 1985, and was published in early 1986. However, it was not referred to in this book, and in fact the only paper which referred to our findings was that of Mukherjee et al in 1987.

The authors referred to a BBC2 Horizon programme which featured both physicians and ME sufferers. They noted, *"There was no escaping the final message: doctors had no answers for ME, so patients must try to help themselves."* In addition they stated that, in 1964, research by Drs Ramsay and Scott had led to the opinion that ME could occur in both endemic and epidemic forms. Those investigators recognised the personal and family tragedies associated with ME and tried to convey this to the medical profession. But in 1970 their work was hindered by the publication of a poorly based claim that Royal Free Disease was simply an outbreak of mass hysteria. Even though the role of hysteria was quickly refuted, the proposal was seized upon by the popular press and the "hypothesis" quickly became a "fact" which dominated medical opinion until the mid-1980s.

Although the title of the book refers to ME, it is of significance that on p 27 there is a stated preference for Chronic Fatigue Syndrome, because, *"...the word chronic makes it clear that the illness is not restricted to a post-viral illness."* The logic behind this claim, as far as ME is concerned, is far from clear. According to the authors, extreme physiological and mental fatigue *"...is the symptom that unites all ME sufferers"* and noted, *"Many diseases manifest themselves with fatigue as one of their symptoms."* (p27) However, there was no discussion about the possible mechanisms of fatigue, nor was there any reference to the views of physiologists who interpret muscle fatigue in terms of inadequate rates of oxygen delivery. It is very unlikely that their claim that, *"ME is unique in that the fatigue is made worse by exercise,"* is sustainable as there is plenty of evidence which shows that the severity of fatigue is increased by strenuous physical activity in many chronic disorders, regardless of the nature of the primary disorder. As far as this aspect is concerned, it seems that investigative journalism lost the will to investigate.

The authors devised a questionnaire based upon 43 questions, *"...not as a means of self-diagnosis, but so you can record exactly the symptoms you are suffering."* This proposal clearly demonstrated the writers' lack of appreciation of the central nervous system dysfunction in ME; manifested as memory problems, and confusion and inability to concentrate.

In a chapter titled, "What causes ME?", the viral theory was discussed at length, followed by the conclusion, "ME may not only be caused by a persistent infection with a virus, but the viral infection may actually damage the body's tissues and metabolism, so that it does not function properly, or take many years to recover." But there is no evidence of tissue damage in ME, and the authors did not explain how remissions might occur if a persistent viral infection was the causal factor. It is much more likely that ME is a dysfunctional state, which may reverse to normal during remissions or increase in intensity during relapses. In their discussion of the relevance of hyperventilation, no reference was made to remissions or relapses.

In a discussion, "What makes ME worse?" (p57) it was stated, *"Severe fatigue and tiredness are the commonest symptoms experienced by people with ME, after a bout of exercise."* While this statement is true, it failed to recognise the body-wide dysfunction which follows over-exertion. In healthy subjects, long-term heavy physical activity is followed by fatigue but with a relatively rapid rate of recovery. In contrast, ME people may take days or weeks to recover from an episode of over-exertion. On p 58, the authors stated, *"...that the muscle metabolism does not follow the normal pathways. This means that lactic acid, a waste product formed during exercise, builds up in the muscle cells"* If lactic acid is formed, this implies that there has been a switch to anaerobic respiration (usually as a consequence of an inadequate rate of delivery of oxygen) so that muscle glycogen is not fully oxidised. Such a sequence described by the authors, is consistent with the physiological concept of fatigue as the result of insufficient oxygen availability. Because an inadequate rate of delivery of oxygen implies impaired capillary blood flow, this situation stimulates the question, "If blood flow to muscles is impaired, do other tissues also suffer inadequate rates of oxygen delivery?"

The authors recognised that, "Every ME sufferer has to learn their own limitations of physical activity," and they noted (p60), "The type of exercise you do, once you feel you are capable, is just as important as how long you do it for. The best things are slow walking or swimming."

Although the possible roles of tea, coffee and alcohol were discussed, it is unlikely that such agents contribute to remissions which may last for days, weeks or even for months. Chapters dealing with allergies and Candida infections serve to illustrate how a simple picture can be complicated. In terms of the Ramsay criteria, which include the absence of positive laboratory tests, the presence of allergies or Candida would exclude a diagnosis of ME.

A failure to recognise the body-wide dysfunction that may occur with ME, resulted in a chapter titled, "The psychological symptoms: anti-depressants, self-help groups and keeping a diary." While the idea of keeping a diary may be good advice, the memory problems associated with cerebral dysfunction could restrict the writing of a diary to "good" days, but the extent of memory problems would also be a factor. In addition, the potential problems of cerebral dysfunction may be the development of "psychological symptoms" and depression. It is very relevant that several studies have shown that depressive illnesses are associated with reduced rates of regional cerebral blood flow. Furthermore, it has been reported that regions of the brain with reduced rates of blood flow during depression show normal rates of blood flow when the depression has resolved. Reduced rates of regional cerebral blood flow have been reported in ME, together with the reduced rates of blood flow in muscles, these findings draw attention to the possibility that impaired blood flow might be the major problem in ME. Such a proposal would be consistent with our published findings since the 1986 report.

The authors stated that while tranquilisers were not recommended, anti-depressants could be helpful. It was suggested that ME sufferers should get in touch with other sufferers or join a Support Group, with the objective of finding out as much as possible about ME.

Chapters 10-12, deal with general aspects of ME, such as employment, benefits, sex and relationships and sleep and rest, while chapters 13-15 discussed various aspects of treatment, noting that anti-viral drugs appeared to be ineffective in ME. Why this could happen if the cause was a persistent viral infection was not discussed. The inconsistent results from studies using gammaglobulin were noted, and a discussion concerning allergies raised the question of whether or not a diagnosis of ME should exclude those with allergies.

Therapies based upon alternative medicine concepts including homeopathy, relaxation, transcendental meditation, biofeedback, self-hypnosis, visualisation, and massage, were discussed, and it was recognised that they lacked scientific support. In the discussion of "Food and ME" (chapter 15), it was recognised that there was no basis for targeting a specific diet, so it not surprising that the authors should conclude, *"ME is still one of the great medical mysteries."*

5. Smith DG. Understanding ME: the phenomena of myalgic encephalomyelitis and acute onset post viral fatigue syndrome. Robinson Publishing, London, 1989, 1991.

Summary. This book could be a source of confusion for ME people, as it is unclear just what the author believes is the relationship between ME and acute onset post viral fatigue syndrome (AOPVFS). As the 1991 copy contains no references to events between 1989 and 1991, it is probably just a reprint. The text lacks any discussion of the possible mechanisms of muscle fatigability, tiredness and malaise, which are considered to be the effects of a viral infection. He believes that AOPVFS is a disease process initiated by a virus, and which is immunologically mediated. Surprisingly, he stated that recovery from AOPVFS was quite predictable, which suggests that he was not working with ME. It is unlikely that ME people will obtain much useful information from this book.

In the introduction, the author recommended that the name ME should be retained in England. However, he stated, *"...the disease process is purely organically and virologically based,"* but on p 90 he wrote, *"This still leaves quite a large proportion of AOPVFS patients in which there is no direct relationship with persistent enterovirus."* So it is not surprising that on p200 he raised the question, *"Are ME and AOPVFS the same disease?"*

While a series of case histories are provided, they do not lead to comments on the cause of fatigue or other symptoms. Given his stated belief that the disease process is organically and virologically based, there is some confusion in the discussion on "What is ME?" He stated, *"ME must clearly contain a number of different disease processes as possible causes. It is then a syndrome rather than a specific diagnosis."* But the Ramsay criteria would reject a diagnosis of ME if "different disease processes" were evident.

The author stated (p22), "The clinical picture of ME is one of fluctuation. Patients can have good days or bad days, good weeks or even months, or even periods of relatively good health extending into years, without ever having quite recovered from their "flu"; they may be struck down at any time by a recurrence of symptoms. Some are remitting, most show a gradual reduction in symptoms." He stated that, "Within ME we are probably working with functional abnormalities of cellular metabolism."

In chapter 3 (p25), he discussed "Acute Onset Post Viral Fatigue Syndrome" and in the following chapter described a study which included a large questionnaire. An interesting aspect was that the results from the questionnaire had a male to female ratio of 1 : 3 which is the same sex ratio reported in a number of ME outbreaks, but this was not remarked upon.

The author discussed virology in chapter 6 (p67). "My feeling is that AOPVFS is a disease process that is initiated by a virus; that the disease process is immunologically determined." Later in answer to the question, "Does anything else cause acute onset post viral fatigue syndrome?", he stated "The answer is emphatically 'No'" However there were other problems and he recognised (p86), "The fact that we can detect it (a virus) in the faeces and in the blood does not necessarily make it pathogenic – but it seems likely that this is the case." However, these statements concerning the pathogenicity of the virus do not sit well with the statement (p90), "This still leaves quite a large proportion of AOPVFS patients in which there is no direct relationship with persistent enterovirus" This statement would seem to indicate that there was a problem in separating ME from AOPVFS.

"Where is the disease and what is going on?" is the title of chapter 8. In discussing muscle weakness, impaired blood flow was not considered, and the problem was considered to be dependent on brain function. There was no clear conclusion about muscle fatigability, nor why activity led to muscle fatigue, but it was noted, (p118), *"In the acute phase of the disorder, the degree of weakness and fatigue varies very rapidly, in some cases, from hour to hour."* There was no comment about how such changes might occur. The work on muscle function in CFS by Lloyd et al was quoted, but the author failed to recognise the different consequences of "static" exercise, as used by Lloyd et al, and those of "dynamic" exercise.

He concluded (p128) that the functional problems related to hypothalamic dysfunction, and that it was possible that a virus maintained the disease, *"...though this may not be true."* In contrast to the findings of Behan et al in Glasgow, no virus was located in the muscles of patients with AOPVFS. Although a list of stressors was incomplete, stress was considered to be, *"...a predisposing factor,"* although what stress did was not discussed.

The contents of chapter 9, "The natural history of AOPVFS," greatly resembles the ME situation. In discussing "How much activity?" it was stated "...*activity in small amounts, in a slow incremental fashion*" just as would be suggested for ME. And the author could be referring to ME when he stated *"From my observations, I am sceptical that if the illness has extended beyond two-and-a-half years, recovery can ever be complete, although there is a tendency to improve, long-term."* Rather surprisingly he stated "...*I have found the rate of recovery of AOPVFS is quite predictable"* but he did not expand on this comment. Although he provided no explanation, on p203 it was recommended that patients should avoid vaccinations. Relatively few alternative treatments were suggested. He considered the Alexander technique, "...*may be helpful for ME sufferers"* and that acupuncture was worth considering. Aromatherapy, reflexology and yoga were mentioned also. It was not considered that Candida played a part in the disorder, and it was stated, *"My disease definition of AOPVFS is that the patients were previously well, and currently have no other particular diseases."* While this is very similar to part of the Ramsay criteria, it needs to be emphasised that according to previous statements, it would include patients with and without evidence of enteroviral infection. This statement seems to compound the confusion concerning the author's concept of AOPVFS, and how it relates to ME, and it certainly does nothing to help in "Understanding ME."

Books Written by Physicians

1. Dawes B, Downing D. Why ME? A guide to combating viral illness, Collins, Glasgow, 1989, 1990.

Summary. For those who suffer from ME and their carers the contents of this book are likely to be a source of confusion. A particular problem arises from the opinions of the authors about how post-viral syndrome relates to ME. As many of their viewpoints are contrary to the opinions of most authors, this divergence can only lead to a lack of clarity. In general there is a lack of scientific explanations for situations which the authors considered to be factual.

As both authors appear to be practitioners of alternative medicine, it is not surprising that their views are different from those of other physicians writing about ME. Throughout the text, post-viral syndrome (PVS) and ME seemed to be used in an interchangeable manner, yet on p1 they stated, *"Both PVS and ME describe the symptoms recorded by the patient, not the cause of the disease."* It is difficult to understand just what that statement was meant to convey. Although the book is titled, "Why ME?" it seems that ME is only a bit player, and on p4 the authors asked, *"Where is the line to be drawn between normal post-viral, or post-traumatic or post-operational and true post-viral syndrome?"* Such a question indicates the rejection of the Ramsay criteria, which would exclude patients with abnormal laboratory findings and evidence of another disease state. Furthermore, to a major extent, the asking of such a question reflects a lack of any attempt to understand the pathophysiology of the problem. Although the authors choose to use the term "fatigue," there is no evidence that they have explored the relevant literature. For example, a 1921 report noted that fatigue could not be defined or measured and proposed that the term fatigue should be absolutely banished from strict scientific discussion.

Even though the variable nature of the symptoms was recognised, there was no attempt to explain how remissions might occur if the cause was a persistent viral infection. The authors state *"However, the major reason for the fluctuations is the persistent drive and determination to over-do-it – so common in ME sufferers."* (p8) Such a proposal implies that the authors have had little contact with ME people, as my experience in meeting with ME groups in six countries does not support their idea. Although the authors discussed muscle weakness in terms of anaerobic respiration, no reasons (such as an inadequate rate of blood flow) were put forward to explain the shift from aerobic respiration. Yet they proposed that a circulatory problem could be the cause of cold hands and feet. In marked contrast to the ME situation, it was stated that depression was rarely a presenting feature in PVS. In contrast to my experience and that of others concerning ME, the authors claimed that 75% to 85% of about 1000 patients *"...are recovering to a significant degree."* (p22)

Given the title of the book, "Why ME?" it seems strange that the reason for writing the book was to increase public awareness of PVS, even though it was not clearly separated from ME.

The situation was not clarified by the establishment of a clinic in 1985, which was, *"...specifically devoted to the nutritional and allergic treatments of PVS and other IMMUNOLOGICAL DISORDERS"* (my capitals) (p29). According to the Ramsay criteria, both allergies and immunological problems would preclude a diagnosis of ME. The possibility that ME patients were not involved seems to be supported by the statement *"Most patients I saw in the first year or two of starting my clinic are now completely well, working full-time and leading exciting and dramatic lives."* I do not know of any similar outcome in other studies of ME. The approach to treatment seemed to have psychosomatic overtones, as an important aspect of treatment involved the changing of lifestyles. The treatment required *"...changing your diets, changing your lifestyle and changing your thought patterns and attitudes"* (p34). It is difficult to link such an approach with the concept of ME as an organic disorder, and this difficulty was reinforced by another statement (p48-9). *"In other words, the multiple malfunctions which make up ME do not descend upon you out of the blue. They have been quietly developing in most cases for months, years, maybe decades."* This very unusual idea would be contrary to the experience of those ME people who had a sudden onset of their disorder.

After a discussion of allergy in PVS, chapter 7 dealt with, "Help from nutrition," and it was stated (p61), "In no area (the lack of essential nutrients) is this more true than in ME, because several different systems of our bodies have gone wrong at the same time, and each of the component problems can make the other ones worse." No supporting evidence was provided, but it is worth noting that multi-system problems would arise if there was a systemic impairment of blood flow. Nor was supporting evidence provided for the rather controversial statement, "People with ME have chronic and often multiple infections." I have never seen a similar claim, but if there were multiple infections, there would be positive laboratory tests which would exclude a diagnosis of ME. And one is led to wonder how remissions could occur during multiple infections.

"Practical Nutritional Therapy," was the title of chapter 8. Although the use of vitamin B12 was discussed, there was no evidence that the authors were aware of the widespread use, in general practices in England, of injections of hydroxocobalamin for the treatment of tiredness. When discussing essential fatty acids, it was not clear that the authors recognised that if the enzyme, delta-6-desaturase was dysfunctional, then it would not be possible to metabolise both omega-3 and omega-6 fatty acids. But a daily supplement of evening primrose oil was recommended for those with ME. My experience with a larger dose of evening primrose oil is that not all patients responded, but there is no statement about their experience with the oil.

Much of the latter part of the book relates to behavioural aspects, and includes some surprising claims. For example, concerning in-patients in psychiatric hospitals, it was stated (p29), *"Only if the psychiatrist agrees have I been able to institute any treatment for their post-viral syndrome, but I think that I can say that all the patients I have seen in this situation have recovered."* If the patients had a psychiatric diagnosis then they would not have ME, but there is no record of the nature of the treatment. Trying to gain some understanding of their approach to the treatment of ME was not made easier by the following statement (p132), *"I have had two patients who experienced dramatic healing within a matter of minutes after they had received prayer for their post-viral syndrome."*

Many behavioural explanations dealing with PVS have little relationship with science, even though they are stated in a factual manner. For example, (p137), *"Many sufferers have come to realise that their post-viral syndrome follows an up and down course (the medical term is relapsing and remitting)."* As a characteristic of ME is a relapsing/remitting course, which has not been shown in any viral infections, it would be more likely that the patients involved had ME rather than PVS. It was proposed that *"…if you deliberately calm down and slow down, then your body will actually begin to recover,"* but what mechanisms would lead to recovery were not discussed. The idea that frustration *"…can lock you into a condition of permanent stress which will cause your immune system to become depressed and non-functioning"* is expressed as a matter of fact on p141.

In a general discussion of the possible inheritance of PVS (p150) it was stated, *"We don't know exactly what kind of illness we are dealing with in post-viral syndrome."* So it is not surprising that two pages later it was stated, *"…it is not simply exposure to the virus or other organism which gave you ME, it was your own weakened defences."* This was followed by the significant conclusion on p153, *"For us, the message is clear: if you have post-viral syndrome, your immune system must be compromised."* It seems that it is over to the reader to separate how the effects of immune system dysfunction lead to either ME or PVS, as the authors have failed to make this clear.

LESLIE O. SIMPSON & NANCY BLAKE

2. Macintyre A. M.E. Post-viral syndrome. How to live with it. Unwin Hyman Limited, London, 1989.

Summary. This book reports the experience of a female physician who fell victim to ME. As the book contains much common sense advice, based upon her personal struggle with ME, it should be read by ME people and carers. When I met Dr. Macintyre in 1995, she was still far from well, eight years after the onset of her disorder. To a major extent it seemed that she preferred PVS to ME, and on p37 noted, "ME seems to be a persistent viral infection," although two pages later she noted the various triggers which set off ME. I was most intrigued by her comments re red blood cells and blood flow, which to a great extent presage my concept of a dysfunctional state resulting from impaired capillary blood flow. However, she seemed not to recognise the significance of her ideas.

Dr. Macintyre was diagnosed as having ME in 1987. In the introduction she stated, "*This book brings together everything that is known so far about ME, and all known ways of coping with it.*" However, it will be shown that there were a number of published reports to which she did not refer. In the early pages she discussed the manifestations of ME, noting the profound exhaustion made worse by exercise, and the expression of a number of bizarre symptoms. Although relapses and remissions were noted, the implications of remissions were not discussed. The author asks (p39) "So, assuming that a variety of viruses, and indeed, other infections and even immunizations trigger off ME, what other factors are involved?" Although she commented on the findings of Mukherjee et al, that four of seven relapsed cases had red cells with abnormal shape, she failed to note that that study was stimulated by the 1986 report of poor filterability of ME blood, by Simpson et al. And there was no acceptance that the changed red cells were of any importance. While the author noted that ME people had problems with poor memory, confusion, slurred speech, word blocks, loss of balance and poor coordination, there was no explanation of this involvement of the central nervous system.

In summing up "What causes ME?" the author considered four possibilities; (a) there is a persistent virus; (b) something has upset the immune system such as a long-past virus or a new virus or environmental factors (pesticides, chemicals); (c) maybe there is an inherited disposition; (d) "physical exhaustion at the time of infection may have an adverse effect."

However, none of those possibilities provide a basis for understanding the nature of a remitting/relapsing disorder. Although Behan's concept that "*ME is a metabolic disorder associated with defective immunoregulation*" was quoted, it was stated also "*There is no single expert who can confidently explain what causes ME, or exactly what is happening in our bodies.*" The author stated (p61), "*The diagnosis still rests on a careful history and exclusion of other conditions.*"

Three patient groups were recognised. One group gradually gets better and stays better. A second group had remissions and relapses, in some cases with remissions lasting for several years. The third group had no remissions and remained unwell. Following a discussion of the various factors known to reduce the function of the immune system, the author made the important point (p71), that her advice was not aimed at curing ME, it was aimed at lessening the severity of symptoms to encourage remissions and to help ME

60

sufferers to live comfortably. To a very great extent her approach is not different from my own, with improving the quality of life being the objective, rather than seeking a cure.

In the following fifty pages, various coping strategies are discussed, and the role of nutrition was examined. Nearly twenty pages were devoted to the use of mineral supplements, which even included a recommendation for the use of germanium, although today its use is contra-indicated.

Although the topics are peripheral to ME, twenty-two pages were allocated to Candida Albicans, eighteen pages to allergies and fifteen pages to chemical sensitivities.

Chapter 12, "Stress and meditation," included the following statement. *"The body cannot remain in a constant arousal by stress, and constantly trying to restabilize, without permanent damage."* However, it would not be easy to find tissue showing stress-related damage, and it is difficult to reconcile permanent damage with the remitting/relapsing nature of ME which is recognised by the author. Later it was stated *"In ME, the viral infection which appeared to trigger it off, may have been the 'last straw', leading to literal exhaustion and collapse."* Rather strangely, this suggestion implies that the viral infection is a secondary factor. Transcendental meditation was considered a useful technique to reduce the effects of stress in ME.

In a discussion on depression (chapter 12), it was stated "Depression is an extent of unhappiness, beyond the point where it can be explained by a cause," and, "Depression affects most bodily functions." The possibility that the factor responsible for altering bodily functions might also cause depression was not considered. In addressing the question, "Why is depression so common in ME?" three possible factors were identified:

> *"(1) All virus infections cause some degree of depression. (2) It is postulated that many ME symptoms may be caused by the continued production of interferon in the body as a response to a persistent virus. (3) If the virus takes up residence in some brain cells, then quite a lot of brain functions are interfered with."* It was concluded (p206), *"So ME depression should therefore be seen as yet another NASTY symptom, rather than to do with the personality of the sufferer."*

From my personal viewpoint, there is no doubt that chapter 16 "Daylight and oxygen" is the most interesting section of the book. On p226, it was stated that, *"…oxygen supply to some tissues in ME seems to be poor, especially during a relapse."* Five reasons for this were given: (1) Poor circulation to the extremities. (2) Small artery muscle tone may be faulty. (3) Small blood vessels may be constricted due to faulty nerve impulses. (4) Reduced blood flow in small vessels as a result of reduced heart output. (5) Night time disorders of breathing regulation. On the following page was this interesting passage:

> *"It is probable that during a relapse, there is something wrong with the red blood cells, making it harder for them to travel along the smallest vessels (capillaries) to supply oxygen to the tissues. Researchers in Australia have examined the blood of patients with the classic features of ME, during and after relapse. The red blood cells become abnormally shaped during a relapse, losing their bi-concave, smooth, disc-like appearance. In this form red cells would be less able to pass through capillaries. This odd appearance had only been observed before in the red blood*

cells of athletes who had just run a marathon. These findings would explain the poor microcirculation and poor oxygenation of tissues, and hence the impaired removal of by-products of metabolism such as lactic acid from the tissues."

While it is true that post-marathon blood had changed red cells, the change was to cupforms (stomatocytes). But there are earlier studies, and in the early 1970s, there were several publications concerning the red cell shape in muscular dystrophy and in 1977 cuptransformation of red cells was reported in Huntington's Disease. Furthermore, as a 1984 paper reported that red cell shape played a role in oxygen uptake and release, it would seem that a change in the shape populations of red cells had physiological implications. However, what was most surprising was to find that in essence, Dr. Macintyre had set out my concept of the pathophysiology of ME, even though there is no indication that she realised the full implications of what she had written. While this could reflect a lack of appreciation of the fundamental importance of normal rates of capillary blood flow, the implications of what she had written had not been apparent in the early chapters, nor was it alluded to in the latter parts of the book.

In chapter 16, "Drugs, dentistry, immunization," it was recommended that no drugs should be taken without having discussed them with a doctor – FIRST! Despite claims of the toxic effects of mercury amalgam fillings, the author recommended that such fillings should not be removed. Even though she would not have known of the effects of immunization on red cell shape, it was stated, (p240) *"Unless it is obligatory before entering a foreign country, the advice to ME patients is DON'T HAVE IMMUNIZATIONS."* Further indications of her lack of recognition of the importance of her concept of the adverse effects of shape-changed red cells on capillary blood flow, are mirrored in her discussion of alternative therapies. (p 255-60) However, it was concluded, *"…in the absence of any organised trials of different therapies for a standardised group of ME patients, any evidence of one treatment being better than another is anecdotal."*

The remainder of the book deals with practical problems, benefits and sources of information and help. Twelve pages were devoted to children and ME, and it was concluded, *"At the moment no one has come up with any magic cure for ME sufferers. The basic principles of management are no different from those advised for adults."*

In her conclusions, Dr. Macintyre emphasised that the term CURE had been avoided, but she made no mention of her concept of pathophysiology which she propounded on p227. So I am left with the opinion that she had failed to recognise the full implications of what she had written.

3. Shepherd C. Living with ME (2nd Edition), Cedar, London, 1992.

Summary. This book contains such an enormous amount of information (most of it relative to sufferers in the UK) that it should be compulsory reading for sufferers and carers AFTER they have read "The mile-high staircase," because in some parts it may be too much for sufferers. Even though Dr. Ramsay was his physician, it seems that Dr. Shepherd has rejected his view that ME should be separated from post-viral fatigue states. Although he referred to one of my papers he erroneously referred to me as "…expert in haematology", which indicated that he failed to recognise that I was working in the field of haemorheology. Rather strangely, he made no reference to our 1986 report, as the finding of poorly filterable blood in ME people seems to have been the first report of an abnormality in ME people.

Possibly because his concept of ME appeared to be rooted in immune dysfunction in a post-viral state, remissions and the adverse effects of physical over-exertion would be inexplicable.

Despite some misgivings about his ideas of the cause of the problem, there is no doubt that the author has put together a vast amount of information based upon his personal experience with ME. It seems important that this information should not be contaminated by references to CFS.

This book records the experiences of a GP who was stricken with ME. On p25 he stated that enteroviruses were considered to be *"the most consistent group of viruses associated with ME."* He recognised that pesticides and vaccinations were other causes, but their mode of action was not discussed. He considered there were three groups of ME people. Group 1 comprised those who, *"...after months or years, make a full or significant recovery and so return to their normal pattern of life."* Group 2 those in this group suffer an erratic disease course of remissions and relapses. During remissions there are periods of *"...relative normalcy,"* then ME returns as the result of another infection, stress or over-activity. Group 3 Patients in this category experience chronic, unremitting ME associated with chronic disablement.

The initial symptoms were those of an ordinary "flu," but most ME patients continued to feel unwell and tired. It was stated (p46) that *"...the cardinal ME symptoms of exercise-induced muscle fatigue and brain malfunction became more and more apparent, and undue stress from an early return to work causes a marked exacerbation."* Any repetitive activity quickly produced weakness, with a very variable recovery time, from minutes to days. On p59 the author noted that oxygen was brought to muscles by red blood cells, and the resulting glycolysis produced energy WHEN OXYGEN AND ENZYMES ARE IN THE CORRECT QUANTITIES. (My emphasis) This implies that if the rate of blood flow was reduced so that the amount of oxygen was less than the correct quantities, then glycolysis would not proceed. McLuskey (his ref 138) was quoted as demonstrating a reduction in the patients' aerobic physical work capacity, but blood flow was not considered as a factor in the muscle dysfunction.

In discussing, "ME and the brain," the author stated "My current view is that the primary disturbance involves a persisting virus," and he noted later "Other factors such as increased lymphokine production and changes in blood flow or energy production may also be playing a part BUT THEY ARE PROBABLY OF SECONDARY IMPORTANCE." (My emphasis) It is difficult to imagine how tissues could function normally in the absence of normal rates of blood flow. The author made no comments relating to how a persisting viral infection could be involved in a remitting/relapsing condition. It was considered that "viral takeover" of neuro-transmitter production (which controlled mood, energy, sleep and well-being) allowed the fatigue of ME to be considered as central, and not peripheral, i.e. in the muscles. This proposal was followed by a discussion of brain malfunction and what patients could do about it.

With regard to cold hands and cold feet, it was stated that tiny blood vessels clamp down, and the problem was worsened by cigarette smoke. It should be noted that cold hands and feet are also reported in other conditions with shape-changed red cells, and that cigarette smoking makes red cells stiffer which increases their resistance to flow. The author advised ME patients not to smoke, as the nicotine constricts the small blood vessels even further.

In commenting about, "ME and your doctor" Dr. Shepherd stated "The current trend towards high-tech medicine has also falsely raised the expectations of many patients, as to what doctors can do in 'curing' disease." Eight pages later he wrote, "So at the present time (1991), there is no reliable, objective way of confirming that someone has ME – it is still down to the doctor's skills and intuition." Other causes of "chronic fatigue" were discussed under headings such as neurological disease, infections, hormonal changes, rheumatic disorders and in other conditions such as alcohol abuse and hypotension. In several of these conditions it has been found that changed red cell shape populations are associated with reduced rates of flow in capillaries.

On p 122 it was stated "People with ME do not make easy patients. You've got what is probably a long-term illness that can't be "cured". So from a GP's point of view, ME people are not the easiest of people to manage successfully." And this opinion was reinforced two pages later "Any sort of cure for ME is a long way off." He noted the frequent problem reported by ME sufferers of finding a helpful doctor, "There isn't any easy answer about how to establish a good doctor/patient relationship: a lot depends on pure luck and where you happen to live."

With regard to "Self-help," he wrote, "A period of slow, steady convalescence is essential – something which has gone out of fashion in modern medicine." Although he stated on p151, that "ME research has already suggested that there are problems with the red cells themselves, as well as a lack of oxygen to vital muscle and nerve cells," the statement does not make it clear that the primary problem is an inadequate rate of delivery of oxygen because of the reduced rate of flow in capillaries, due to poorly deformable red cells.

In noting that *"Some ME patients experience quite a severe reaction or relapse in symptoms following vaccinations"* Dr. Shepherd would be unaware that there is a dramatic change in red cell shape populations after vaccinations, and such changes would be additive to any pre-existing changes in red cell shape.

Fifty pages of text were devoted to alternative and complementary approaches to treatment, and the use of supplements. This was followed by about fifty pages of advice to patients and carers living in England, and carers and relatives were advised to find out all they could about ME, in order to be of maximum assistance to the sufferers. Helpful advice was offered on how ME people should handle their job and what they could do to increase their mobility. Information about sources of help and about the availability of additional benefits was provided also.

4. Natelson BH. Facing and fighting fatigue. A practical approach. Yale University Press, New Haven, 1998.

Summary. Although there are many aspects of this book which are open to challenge, the objective is to gain some enlightenment about the problems ME people have in finding a sympathetic doctor, and Professor Natelson has provided that information.

While the topic of the book is of general interest (rather than being applicable to ME people), the chapter, "Understanding the doctor," is of particular relevance. What he has written will allow ME people to understand why they have to search for a sympathetic doctor, because in his view, doctors are moulded by the curriculum. In a paragraph titled "The moulding process" (p94) it is stated:

> *"The medical student who is focussed and mature can avoid moulding. Unfortunately, the youth and relative inexperience of most medical students makes them highly susceptible to peer pressure that changes a considerate young doctor-to-be into someone who can be described by the 3 Bs, - brash, boorish and bullying – in addition to being unkind and a poor listener."*

Further down the page he wrote:

> *"Except for the rare young doctor who realises that the whole is more important that its parts, and has both the time and the intelligence to put the pieces together to better understand the whole patient, most young doctors think it adequate to know only the facts of medicine. Thus the curriculum forces into the student a bias in favour of technology and against communication and empathy."*

This critical appraisal follows on p 97 "Thus medical materialism joins the other forces that mould the young doctor into someone who does not hear what the patient is saying," and on the following page:

> *"Doctors' ears tend to perk up when they hear what they expect, and drop when what they hear means nothing to them. Again this reflects what they have been taught." "Something that is of major importance to the patient is not heard by the doctor. Instead the doctor continues trying to get information that makes medical sense to him or her. And once again, if the doctor cannot make medical sense out of the history, he or she assumes that the problem is psychological, that there is nothing wrong with the patient and that the patient should not be wasting the doctor's time. The patient is left to figure out what to do next."*

ME people should be very grateful to Professor Natelson for providing a basis for understanding the nature of the unsympathetic doctor.

The end of Dr. Simpson's reviews of books dealing with ME, including some by people who have ME, is perhaps an appropriate point at which to continue my story.

Going Back To Work - My New Job

After I had been sick with ME for a few weeks, I experimented with going back to work at the Centre. I found that I couldn't sit up at the table around which we held the morning and evening de-briefing sessions, and lying on a bean bag didn't facilitate participation in the discussions. After two hours I was exhausted to the point of weeping, and gave up the attempt. It seemed that returning to work full-time at the Centre was not going to become a possibility, or not for a very long time.

It was my great good fortune that I had become friends with April Henry, whose husband, Fred, was one of the Assistant Directors of the Humberside Social Services Department. Fred was sympathetic to my situation, and firmly believed that with a sufficiently challenging job, my health would return. The Principal Officer Health for Grimsby and Scunthorpe was going off on maternity leave, and I was offered the opportunity to interview for the post.

One of my most vivid memories to do with being ill was trying to get to the interview. I can't remember whether I was driven to a near-by spot, and I had not yet decided that a wheelchair would improve my life. The picture and the physical memory is of trying to walk down a narrow, unfamiliar pathway, whilst feeling frightened that I wasn't going to make it.

I must have – I got the job, and it was ideal.

The Principal Officer, Health, was an advisory post which was mainly concerned with the planned transfer of care for mentally ill, mentally handicapped and the elderly from long-stay hospitals run by the NHS into community care facilities run by the Social Services Departments. The job consisted of going to meetings and writing reports. My son and his friends, who had driving licenses but no jobs (this being Hull, in the 80's) were willing to be paid volunteers' expenses for driving me from Hull to Grimsby or Scunthorpe and wheel-chairing me to meetings. The job included a mileage allowance, and a telephone allowance. The Finance Officer, Tony Murphy, very kindly provided me with an obsolete PC. The telephone allowance and the PC made it possible to do a lot of organising of my time and activities from in bed, or lying down on a settee.

Attending meetings could be a problem, especially on the occasional times when I had to drive myself. On the morning of a one-day workshop which I was presenting at the hospital in Scunthorpe, my driver failed to arrive. He wasn't on the phone, and I couldn't risk waiting and being late. Not only did I have to drive the exhausting, twisting road which was the shortest route to the hospital, I then had to carry boxes of papers into the building. At noon, there was a long walk to the dining facilities, where I lay down for half an hour, hoping to be well enough to get back and continue the afternoon. Completely done in, I had to ask to be taken back to the workshop room in a wheelchair. Somehow I managed to lead the afternoon activities, and drive myself back to Hull. I was in bed for three weeks after that but fortunately it had been at the beginning of the Christmas period, so I didn't have to take much time off sick.

Sometime during this period I realised that I had begun to feel phobic about going to meetings at the Scunthorpe Area Headquarters. Usually I was dropped off in a tiny side street about fifty feet from the entrance, and although going up to the first floor where the offices were was a bit of a challenge, I could usually manage. Trying to figure out why I had started to feel panicky about meetings there, I recalled a day when I had had to drive myself. The only parking lot was about five hundred feet from the office, and I had had the usual decision to make about where best to park. Accessing nearby spaces usually required a certain amount of exhausting manoeuvring. Parking in an easier space further away meant a longer walk, whilst carrying a handbag and papers for the meeting, and I could never feel sure of being able to manage the longer distance. On this particular day, I had left the car, started walking toward the office, and realised that there was no way on earth I could go any farther, even though I was only about five hundred yards from my destination. I sat down on the kerb, frustrated and despairing. Here I was, supposedly a successful, professional woman, reduced to sitting helplessly in the street, like someone who had no other home. Even had someone offered to help, I was still unable to walk the needed distance, and they couldn't very well carry me. After a few minutes in this state of utter humiliation, attracting disapproving stares from the many passers-by, I realised that there was a taxi stand nearby. The driver was bemused, but managed to sound sympathetic, as he drove me a mile around the one-way system in order to get me to a place that was just a couple of hundred yards from where I had accosted him. I got to the meeting, but the stress, despair, and humiliation I had felt took its toll, and, remembering this event, I realised why had begun to fear that place. This illustrates how a genuinely psychiatric symptom, 'irrational' feelings of panic, can arise as a result of situations caused by physical effects of the illness, and once I remembered the event, the panic evaporated.

Wheelchair

At some point in the midst of the logistical and the psychological stresses and strains of my job I decided to get a wheelchair. I don't remember exactly when I acquired it but I do remember the shocked reaction from my boss (one of the Humberside Social Services Assistant Directors). 'Are you trying to commit career suicide?' was his horrified response. Notwithstanding that this was the Social Services Department: the Department that cares for people who are disabled, ill and/or elderly! I was later told that of all the local government departments, social services departments are the least tolerant of disability in their staff.

The wheelchair was amazingly liberating because it greatly expanded my range of possibilities. It was a transit model, the one with smaller wheels that is designed to be pushed by someone else. For someone disabled by ME, wheeling one of those self-propelled ones using one's own arms would take just as much physical effort as walking around, thus defeating the purpose. When I was still very ill, I needed to have someone with me to fold the wheelchair up, put it in the car, unload and unfold it at the other end, and push me around in it. Having thus conserved energy, I would then be able to get up to look at clothes on a rail, or walk around a shop a little bit, as well as get to the meetings that were the main part of my job. It was very restricting always having to find someone who was available to help me out, but at least I had people who were willing and kind. And I know this makes a critical difference to the quality of the experience. It can be quite a lot of fun if you're with someone who likes you and likes doing it. The experience of being pushed around begrudgingly is very demoralising.

I loved my wheelchair because it represented freedom and it gave me a way of re-entering the world. But in a wheelchair, you are caught up in a network of negative social assumptions and these can be hard to counter. For example, people tend to assume that you must be completely disabled, that you will look dowdy, that you are unhappy, that you are in pain and that you are not very bright. Above all, you will be regarded as someone who is asexual. Oh, and curious children must be shushed immediately, "Don't ask that lady what's wrong with her, that's dreadfully rude" But why should children not have things explained to them? Disability is an important subject, and a friendly explanation may help defuse a child's anxieties, at least by learning that a person in a wheelchair can still be friendly and articulate.

The very first time I tried it out, I had the experience of being invisible. My husband ran into one of his university colleagues when we had gone to meet our son who was returning from Holland on the North Sea Ferry. This man proceeded to have a conversation with Tony, without the slightest attempt to include me (although come to think of it, that might have happened even if I hadn't been in a wheelchair!).

I decided that wheelchairs should be designed with reference both to their function as a vehicle (motorbike stickers, tribal decals) and their function as fashion accessory (changeable colours to match your outfit, and your eye-shadow.) This idea has not yet been taken up by the industry, but it should be. Not everyone in a wheelchair is 85, or thinks their life is over. Or is celibate!

And My Dog

One evening, in the exertion-limited pursuit of pleasure, I was sitting in the wheelchair out in front of the house, waiting for a friend to pick me up and take me to the nearby club where my son's band was playing. My dog Muttley, best described as a collie on very short legs, was waiting with me. Muttley was never very interested in balls, or dog toys, but he adored sticks. That night while we were waiting he brought me a stick, offering a tugging game. When I took hold of it, the wheelchair started moving decisively down the path propelled by Muttley who was gripping the stick in his teeth and running backwards. We were nearly all the way to the nightclub when my lift finally appeared.

That began a collaboration that gave me another degree of freedom. Whenever I was well enough, or had help to load the wheelchair into the car, I could go around town on my own, with Muttley's assistance. At that time, my family found it terribly embarrassing. Seeing-Eye dogs were acceptable, but the concept of a dog as a disability aide was still unheard of at that time. And the fact that this remained a game, with Muttley running backwards, pulling me along by something held in his teeth, did look very strange. But he could navigate me at speed in a crowded railway station, directed by my hand gestures, and never run into to anyone.

He even helped me get to a meeting in London, on my first unaccompanied expedition outside of Hull. I felt rather silly and neurotic, paying a train fare so that I could have my dog with me. However, the meeting was being held a mile from King's Cross and it coincided with a one-day strike by London Underground staff, which meant at least a two-hour wait for a taxi. With a little help from a solicitous passer-by to get up the initial slight slope just west of King's Cross, Muttley got me to the meeting on time!

The Executive Chair

Unless I could lean back and rest in my chair at work, I would quickly become unable to understand or remember what I was supposed to be doing. I had to fight for an executive chair, the kind that has nice upholstery and a high back, with the facility to tip it backwards into a slightly resting position. These were the prerogative only of people (men, of course) higher up on the pecking order than I was. However, a special concession was made and I was allocated an executive chair. With the aid of this chair it became possible to function in the office, for limited periods.

When the maternity leave of the woman I was covering was at an end, she only wanted to return half-time, and I was offered (with some trepidation) the possibility of becoming the Department's first 'AIDS Officer'. No, I did not want to become the 'AIDS Officer', but I would find it very interesting if I were allowed to become the 'HIV Information and Policy Officer'.

So I continued to cover Grimsby as Principal Officer Health, half-time, and became the HIV Information and Policy Officer for the other half. When I moved from both of these posts to become Senior Social Worker in the Hospital Social Work Team at Castle Hill Hospital, I agreed only on the basis that The Chair came with me. This was both promised and ignored. Before I had formally left, one of my male colleagues ('friends') had removed The Chair to his office. Rather than utter futile protests, I launched a night raid with the help of one of my young informal assistants, and we removed The Chair, under cover of darkness, to the office of the Senior Social Worker at Castle Hill Hospital where it served me faithfully and well until my retirement in 1989.

Life After The Social Services

It was the late 1980s, and a property-buying frenzy was underway. Property in Hull was among the cheapest in the country and, as properties were doubling in value over a short period, speculators were coming up from London and buying up whole streets in Hull as investments.

Tony's generosity enabled me to join this frenzy, and I found out how easy it was to purchase cheap property in the wrong end of town, ending up with four. My plan was to tenant the houses with people who had problems in order to try and run my own mini version of Pashby House. I moved into one of the properties, after a period of living in flats nearer the Park Avenue house. This was the beginning of several chaotic years in which I fulfilled quite a lot of my teen-aged fantasies of bohemian living. The details of this period of my life might serve as a comic novel, or as an account of a noble effort to Do Good for people with problems, or even as an expose by the News of the World into the darker side of a mid-life crisis. In whatever way I choose to frame them the fact remains that they were undeniably an object lesson in how not to make money as a landlady!

I didn't get rich but I did learn a number of valuable lessons, not least that it might be good idea to take other people's advice occasionally. I now know that running a business requires a financial plan, notably absent from my arrangements. It also requires professional help rather than the ad hoc involvement of friends and acquaintances. Location, location, location is more than just a silly mantra! In a neighbourhood where many young people had little education and no prospects, the entrepreneurial spirit so valued in the Thatcher years often took the form of drug-dealing and burglary, to which some of my more enterprising tenants added unannounced departure from furnished accommodation, accompanied by much of the furniture. Hence, Doing Good, in my situation came to require considerable back-up from friends, workmen, Social Services and occasionally the police.

Throughout this time, it is not surprising that I continued to be very ill. Even the legitimate demands of being a responsible landlady were completely beyond me, and I was gradually able to divest myself of the houses, but only with considerable financial help from my mother and brother and a certain amount of good luck.

Eventually, as Tony had met his second wife, and moved with her to Australia, I moved back to Park Avenue to manage it as a multi-occupied property. There were complications similar to those I had experienced with my own houses, but with the support of my assistant, Helen, and my friend, Sue, these were gradually dealt with. I continued to work as a psychotherapist and teach piano there for several years. When, in 2005, the house was sold, I moved, with Sue and her son, Ethan, into our current address, a house owned by the person who bought Park Avenue. I continue to teach piano and work as a psychotherapist.

Now, back to Dr. Simpson....

CHAPTER III
- THE HISTORICAL BACKGROUND TO ME

With the aim of providing a better perspective and appreciation of ME as a health problem, it is proposed that much could be gained from an examination of the history of the disorder. With that objective in mind, this section will address the topic under three headings: namely Pre-ME; ME; and Post-ME. In this way it should become clear why it is necessary to introduce Ramsay's Disease (ME) in order to separate those who suffer from ME from other more inclusive diagnoses.

The Pre-ME period

What follows has been extracted from two main sources. Firstly, the paper by A.D. Acheson, "The clinical syndrome variously called benign myalgic encephalomyelitis, Iceland Disease and epidemic neuromyasthenia," published in 1992, in the book edited by Hyde, Goldstein and Levine, and secondly, the second edition of Ramsay's book, "Myalgic encephalomyelitis and post viral fatigue states" published in 1988.

Acheson's article set out to review the reports of a number of obscure illnesses which began with an epidemic outbreak in Los Angeles in 1934. He noted the variety of names which had been applied to the different outbreaks, so it is worth noting that Hyde has listed no fewer than seventy-eight diagnostic terms which have been applied to the different outbreaks. For this reason it is not surprising that Acheson should note *"The difficulties in defining a disorder from which no deaths have occurred, and for which no causative or toxic agent has been discovered, are obvious."*

The possibility that a single disorder was involved was not supported by the variations in attack rates, according to gender, in the Los Angeles, Iceland, Royal Free Hospital and Punta Gorda outbreaks. The related male/female ratios were 1:4, 1:1.6, 1:3.7. and 1:2.1. In contrast, in the outbreaks in Adelaide, Australia, Dalston, England and Tapanui, New Zealand, 1:1 ratios were reported. In the one hundred ninety-six cases in the Los Angeles epidemic, sixty-nine symptoms were listed, with headache, myalgia and paresis (slight or incomplete paralysis) being the most frequent. In addition there were other symptoms and signs of damage to the brain, spinal cord or peripheral nerves, which were accompanied by mental symptoms relating to memory and confusion. If fever was present it was usually below 100 degrees F. In general, the results from cerebrospinal fluid investigations were predominantly normal. Although relapses were noted to occur in most outbreaks, there was little comment concerning remissions.

There was some doubt expressed about the involvement of a single factor which was related to the incubation periods of a prodromal disorder. While in most outbreaks this was about four days, in the Durban and the Middlesex Hospital epidemics, the incubation time was two to three weeks. In several outbreaks, poliomyelitis was a confusing factor, but this did not apply to the Middlesex Hospital, Bethesda, Royal Free Hospital, Berlin and Punta-Gorda outbreaks.

In the hospital outbreaks there was an unexplained prevalence of nurses, but in five institutional outbreaks there was no evidence that nurses had been infected by staff. In eight of nine outbreaks, it was concluded that the agent responsible was not water- or food-borne. With regard to the clinical features, Acheson noted *"An exact numerical comparison of symptoms and signs, reported in the various outbreaks is not possible."*

There was considerable variation in the modes of onset of the different epidemics. In Los Angeles and in the Royal Free Hospital epidemic, most cases experienced a sudden onset of their symptoms, while in Iceland, neck and back pain were the main problems for the first few days. Of the nineteen cases in New York, fifteen had an insidious onset, while the other four cases had an abrupt onset of their illness. In Adelaide, most patients experienced an abrupt onset, with headaches and a stiff neck. In both the Middlesex Hospital and Berlin outbreaks, most cases had an abrupt onset, while in the Coventry and Punta Gorda epidemics, most patients had an insidious onset of their symptoms. Prodromal symptoms were a feature of the Durban and Bethesda outbreaks.

The basis of this variability in mode of onset and symptomatology remains unexplained. While it is possible that some of the patients involved in these epidemics could have ME, the degree of variation in the mode of onset gives rise to the possibility that different causal agents could be involved. No consideration was given to the possibility that the variation in the way the illness presented might indicate individual variation in susceptibility. The extent of the similarities and differences in the responses to a putative infection may be assessed from the consideration of the different outbreaks.

(a) Los Angeles. Acheson emphasised the importance of Gilliam's account of the fully developed disease in Los Angeles, as it was written without knowledge of subsequent epidemics. Gilliam reported that 94% of cases experienced severe, generalised headaches; 66% had stiffness of the neck or back; pain in muscles was almost a constant feature, but the pain varied in location and intensity from day to day. In addition, the intensity of the pain was aggravated by exertion. In many cases opiates were needed to provide pain relief. Many cases suffered from muscle tenderness, which required the use of cradles to keep the weight of bed clothes off the skin. Muscle twitching and cramps were common complaints. When fever was present, in most cases it was less than 100 degrees F. In about 80% of cases, there was localised muscle weakness, which, like the muscle pain, varied in site and intensity from day to day. In nineteen cases, muscle weakness was noted in the first fourteen days, and in half of these had cleared in four weeks and a further 25% had cleared at eight weeks. Urinary retention was a problem for 12% of cases, and 30% manifested mental symptoms. Gilliam noted

The emotional upsets reported are difficult to interpret. They varied in degree from relatively slight displays of irritability and impatience, to violent manifestations of dislike for people they formerly liked. A common type of upset consisted of crying spells resulting from no known provocation......Other disturbances consisted of loss of memory and difficulty in concentration.

After a course of six to eight weeks, the illness abated, the paresis disappeared in most cases, and the average stay in hospital was about eight weeks.

Ramsay discussed some later reports on the status of some of those involved in the Los Angeles epidemic, without obtaining any evidence for the possible cause of the outbreak. However, he noted that after fourteen years, about 10% of patients reported residual muscle pain, fatigue and mental changes.

On the basis of the information provided, it is difficult to accept that the Los Angeles epidemic is related to ME. However, Ramsay reached the conclusion that *"The outbreak in the Royal Free Hospital in 1955 was an almost exact replica of the outbreak in Los Angeles."*

(b) Iceland. Between 1945 and 1949, one hundred seventy-one males and two hundred ninety-four females, (male to female ratio 1 : 1.7) developed a disorder marked by neck and back pain which was considered to be an outbreak of epidemic neuromyasthenia. After an estimated incubation period of about four days and the development of a low fever, a few days later, limb pain developed. According to Acheson *"Emotional lability, irritability, depression and lack of concentration appeared in convalescence and were extremely troublesome."* In mild cases the disease persisted for from two to four weeks, but more severe cases were unwell for two to three months. However, Ramsay has drawn attention to a study by a neurologist of thirty-nine patients (8.3%) which showed that only about 25% of the more severely affected cases had recovered completely. Many of those patients still exhibited a variety of symptoms, which included fatigability of muscles, muscle pain and loss of memory. In addition, while 44% of mildly affected patients had recovered completely, the remainder continued to be symptomatic.

(c) Adelaide. Acheson referred to this outbreak as an acute illness of short duration which was followed by severe headaches with a mild generalised aching of muscles which cleared after a few days. Some cases suffered urine retention. About four to eight weeks after the original illness, there was a re-appearance of symptoms which included hyperacusis, depression and fatigue. The course of the illness was prolonged and difficult to treat. However, Ramsay painted a very different picture in noting, *"...the stream of paralytic poliomyelitis cases ceased abruptly and were replaced by cases of ME."* While the cerebro-spinal fluid of poliomyelitis cases showed the usual changes, in the ME cases, no cerebro-spinal fluid changes were observed. By April 1951, seven hundred cases had been admitted to hospital, and the male: female ratio was 1: 1. Although it was claimed that a Coxsackie Group B virus was the most likely cause of the inhibition of the poliomyelitis virus, no virus was isolated. At the post mortem examination of monkeys which had been inoculated with human material, it was observed that, *"...minute red spots were found along the sciatic nerves."* Microscopic study revealed white cell infiltration of nerve roots and patchy damage to myelin sheaths. Ramsay suggested that *"This pathological picture of mild, diffuse changes corresponds closely to what might have been expected from clinical observation of patients with neurological involvement in ME."* However he did not define the criteria he had used to decide that ME was involved. And if ME was involved, how could remissions occur if tissue damage was demonstrable?

(d) Middlesex. Hospital Patients in this outbreak reported severe upper body muscle pain, with an apparently mild involvement of the central nervous system. Following these prodromal symptoms, nine of fourteen cases reported a sudden onset of pain, tenderness, spasm and paresis in a limb or limbs. Urinary retention and incontinence were prominent features, and although there were emotional upsets in the acute phase, this did not occur during convalescence. In the majority of cases, by the end of the third week, most of the pain had disappeared, although in a few cases, relapses occurred in the second and third week.

(e) Coventry. Neither Acheson nor Ramsay provided information about the numbers of cases in this outbreak, which occurred in nurses who worked in wards dealing with poliomyelitis patients. The illness had an insidious onset and was marked by headache and neck pains. This was followed by muscle weakness and pain, which did not appear to have been severe. Some cases recovered within a month, and in all cases recovery was substantially complete within two months. Convalescence was characterised by memory problems and a lack of concentration.

(f) Bethesda. While Acheson considered this outbreak to resemble the situation in Coventry, Ramsay pointed out that the author of the report considered that it resembled the Los Angeles epidemic. There were two outbreaks, the first occurring in July 1953, while the second, which was associated with an intake of nurses on August 31, showed the first symptoms on September 18. In total, fifty nurses were involved in a "minor" illness, marked by malaise, headache and low grade fever, which preceded paresis by four to six days. If this stage exceeded six days then gastrointestinal symptoms (diarrhoea, nausea, vomiting) became prominent. The "major" illness was manifested as exacerbations of headache and back stiffness, accompanied by numbness in one or more limbs. While low fevers were common, afternoon temperatures were usually higher than morning temperatures. Acheson noted *"Nervousness, unprovoked crying spells, difficulty in concentration, undue irritability and anxiety occurred in nineteen of twenty six patients studied in detail."* Although twelve of fifty cases were re-examined five months later (in December 1953), none had recovered. All had suffered relapses, some of which related to physical exertion. Other causes of relapses were changes in ambient temperature or the onset of menstruation, and were accompanied by coldness in the lower extremities.

(g) Alaska and Berlin. These outbreaks, which were marked by muscle and limb pain, together with a variety of the symptoms recorded in other outbreaks, were discussed very briefly.

(h) Durban. In February, 1955, fifty-nine nurses became ill within a week, and during the next few weeks another thirty-nine nurses became unwell. While some of the nurses lived in the hospital, some did not. However, there was no spread to patients or to other staff. For up to about two weeks prior to the acute phase, severe occipital headache was the major symptom, but was accompanied by a variety of other symptoms including lassitude, sore throat and painful eyes. There were ten cases of urine retention, and mental symptoms were prominent, including emotional instability and defects in memory and in concentration. While the majority of patients improved in two months, relapses continued for six to nine months and eleven cases were still disabled after three years.

(i) Royal Free Hospital. According to Ramsay, between July 13 and November 24, 1955, two hundred ninety-two of various staff categories were victims of an infectious agent, but only twelve inpatients developed the disease. Of this total, two hundred fifty-five were admitted to hospital, while the remainder were either treated at home or admitted to other hospitals. Acheson noted that it was not possible to separate those symptoms which occurred early from those which occurred later. However, Ramsay noted *"The earliest symptoms were malaise and headache, frequently associated with disproportionate depression and emotional lability."* As had been noted in other outbreaks, a low fever was common. The main cause for concern was pain, sometimes very severe, in the limbs and upper body, which varied in intensity from day to day, or even within the same day. During the second and third week many of the patients became severely ill. For unexplained reasons, ninety-two cases were omitted from the analysis.

> It has always been my understanding that Dr. Ramsay himself had eliminated these ninety-two cases from his analysis because he believed they were psychological, and that it was from inspection of the records **of these patients, only**, that McEvedy and Beard came to the conclusion that the whole outbreak had been an example of 'mass hysteria'.

Of the two hundred cases analysed, one hundred and forty eight showed objective evidence of central nervous system involvement. It was noted that "The neurological manifestations formed a characteristic picture that distinguishes this disease from other infections of the nervous system." But no evidence was presented to support the claim of an infection of the nervous system. While six cases developed depression, major symptoms of sleep problems, uncontrollable weeping, and memory problems, these could be manifestations of a dysfunctional nervous system, rather than a system damaged by an infection. Yet Acheson stated "Cranial nerve LESIONS (my emphasis) occurred in sixty nine of the fully documented cases." In contrast, Ramsay was less specific and stated, "There was a heavy involvement of the cranial nerves." Motor weakness in the limbs was noted in one hundred and two patients, while sensory disturbances occurred in eighty-two cases. Ramsay concluded, "The clinical impression was of a disease producing a diffuse disorder of the nervous system, with a combination of irritative and paralytic signs, WHICH WERE FREQUENTLY TRANSIENT" (my emphasis) The idea of a transient disorder of the nervous system seems to be at odds with the idea of "... infections of the nervous system" and stimulates the question of what type of event causes transient changes. Rather strangely, neither Ramsay nor Acheson provided any information about the development of symptoms, convalescence and recovery of those who were victims of the epidemic

(j) Punta Gorda. In the spring of 1956, there were at least one hundred fifty cases of a disorder for which no causal agent was identified, in a community of two thousand five-hundred residents. The illness occurred in young and middle-aged people; was more severe in females and ran a prolonged, relapsing course. Between May 24 and June 6, 1956, twenty-one patients with similar manifestations of the illness were interviewed. Seventeen of these were female and the ages of those involved ranged from twelve to sixty years. It was stated that the patients had been noting vague symptoms for from one to sixty five days. Fatigue coupled with headache, neck pain, nausea and vomiting were the most frequent symptoms, although nineteen experienced depression and memory problems. Acheson considered that *"It seems that the illness in Punta Gorda ran a sub-acute rather than an acute course, and that objective evidence of disease was minimal."* But Ramsay noted

> *The follow-up examination after five months showed that the course was an irregular one with periods of improvement interrupted by exacerbations of symptoms, often related to physical exertion. The paucity of physical findings in relation to symptoms was striking.*

In summarising the major features of the epidemic outbreaks discussed by Acheson, it seems that the most important finding is the variability in mode of onset and symptomatology, even though there are overall similarities in the outbreaks. Although it was noted in several reports that relapses were triggered by physical exertion, the onset of menstruation and by cold temperatures, there was no discussion of what this implied. From my point of view, it seems that those triggers could provide a key to understanding at least some part of the nature of the disease; i.e. because all three factors have been associated with changes in the shape populations of red cells.

Ramsay made reference to eight outbreaks not discussed by Acheson, and in general there was no obvious deviation from the general pattern observed in other outbreaks. Therefore it is of interest that in his comments on the Finchley outbreak, Ramsay stated *"An outbreak of ME occurred in Finchley in 1964 and continued for two years."* This was the second occasion where Ramsay has referred to "ME" and he stated also

> *A diagnosis of ME was never considered unless most of the following features were present: low grade fever and headache; blurred vision and diplopia; stiff neck; vertigo with a positive Romberg test; nausea and/or vomiting; lymphadenopathy; lower costal or generalised muscular weakness, unrelieved by rest; insomnia and/or vivid dreams, often in colour; frequency or retention of urine; degrees of deafness or hyperacusis.*

It is surprising that the problems of memory and confusion were not considered to be features of ME.

In the Great Ormond Street Hospital for Sick Children outbreak in 1970-71, one hundred forty-five people, mainly nurses, became unwell. The usual "protean symptomatology" noted in other outbreaks were recorded and ten or eleven of the commonest symptoms were similar to those of the Royal Free Hospital epidemic. In addition *"...rapid fatigability on exercise was noted."* At least twenty-eight cases experienced symptomatic relapses with intervals varying from two months to six months, and such a relapsing pattern persisted for several years after the onset of the illness.

Between January 1980 and June 1983, twenty-two patients living in West Kilbride, Ayrshire, were assessed for suspected ME. Sixteen were female and the male to female ratio was 1: 2.7. The female ages ranged from eight to fifty three years and the male ages were from ten to forty one years. The disorder presented as either an acute or a sub-acute illness with a variety of symptoms which included chest pain, sleep disorders and sleep disturbance. Ramsay noted *"Once the disease was established, the most characteristic symptom was extreme exhaustion, particularly after exercise. The exhaustion also occurred after emotional or mental strain."* There was no discussion of what pathological factor or factors could be stimulated by physical or mental activity. What made the West Kilbride cases exceptional was the fact that eighteen of the twenty-two patients were shown to have elevated neutralising antibodies to Coxsackie B virus, and twelve of these had symptoms which persisted for at least six months. Ramsay stated *"Consequently, I had long harboured a suspicion that the triggering factor in ME is to be found in the immunological state of the patient, and research is showing this to be the case."* But if this is the case, then why did six of Coxsackie B-positive patients not have a persisting illness?

In Balfron, Stirlingshire, a general practitioner was stimulated by the events in West Kilbride to make further investigations of his patients with *"...protracted or atypical illnesses."* Twenty patients with suspected ME were selected for virological studies. The results were similar to those of the West Kilbride cases, but were significantly different from those of a normal adult group. When the investigators extrapolated their results to the population at large, they concluded, *"...then there are a large number of ill and unhappy patients in the community and it is suspected that many of these are to be found among returning attenders at medical and psychological clinics."*

The events in Kilbride and Balfron led to a similar study in Helensburgh, where eighty-one cases characterised by multisystem symptomatology were investigated between 1978 and August 1983. Significantly-raised antibody titres to Coxsackie B Group viruses were found in thirty-eight cases (47%) and six others had borderline titres. It was noted that *"The illness bore a close resemblance to descriptions of ME ...and the disease ran a fluctuating course of relapse and remission over many months and even persisted for several years."* The Helensburgh practitioners continued to find new cases *"... with no sign of a fall in incidence."* With a considerable degree of insight, they observed that most reports concerned epidemics rather than the endemic pattern of the cases they had studied.

In concluding, Ramsay wrote *"That observation conforms with the findings of Dr. Betty Scott and myself that the disease is primarily endemic."* What has yet to be shown is the mechanism by which an endemic disorder is transformed into epidemics with very unusual features. Nor is it clear why more than half of those suffering from multisystem symptomatology were negative to Coxsackie B viruses. One is left with the conclusion that Coxsackie B viruses are only one of the triggering agents.

Acheson included in his paper an interesting section titled "Status of patients on discharge from hospital." In the Los Angeles epidemic, the average time to return to duty was 13.6 weeks, but this calculation was based on less than 50% of all cases, as 55% were still on the sick list. In eighteen of forty-three cases there was still definite, localised, and moderate to severe paresis. Gilliam considered that it was not possible to provide an accurate estimate of recovery rates.

Six months after the appearance of the last case in Durban, fifty of ninety-eight nurses had returned to duty with no apparent sequelae and thirty-two were on duty with "...*mild or more serious residua.*" Seven cases were still on sick leave with serious sequelae and the same number was either on vacation or had resigned. Two cases had relapsed and had been re-admitted. In the mild cases, there was full recovery of muscle power within a few days, and convalescence, which was marked by headaches, aching and fatigue, was complete within a month. In contrast, it was three or four months before moderate cases returned to normal, while severe cases were still relapsing up to seven months from the onset of their illness.

The Royal Free Hospital record showed that 57% of cases had less than one month as in-patients, while 28.5% required one to two months of in-patient care. Another 7.5% were in-patients for two to three months and 7% were in hospital for more than three months. Acheson noted "*Convalescence was very prolonged ....and extreme fatigue and general aches and pains made the rehabilitation period extremely tedious and long.*" Those patients who had been on bed rest for more than a month, required six weeks of convalescence before discharge. After convalescence, many nurses could work for only four hours a day. Two years after the onset of the epidemic, four patients still exhibited marked disability.

Of those patients in the Middlesex Hospital outbreak, seven of fourteen cases had no physical signs when they were discharged, on average, one month after the onset, while the remainder exhibited a variety of symptoms.

In a section titled, "The aftermath – relapses" Acheson noted that in all outbreaks, except that in Coventry, relapses were a feature of the illness. He stated that in five outbreaks "...*relapses or exacerbation of symptoms in women, have coincided with menstrual periods.*" In addition, physical exertion or cold weather was also associated with relapses. The time between relapses was very variable. Acheson cited a comment by Galpine and Brady which stated that after a period of perfect health in the interim of three years, a second relapse occurred. Relapses could involve regions previously affected or could involve new regions, and Acheson wrote "*There appeared to be no predisposing cause for them, although in many cases they were associated with untimely over-exertion, or with some phase, usually the onset of menstruation.*" During cold, damp weather, there was increased pain and a sense of ill-being in those who did not suffer a recrudescence of symptoms.

In summarising, "The sub-acute and chronic stages" the author pointed out that in general, most of the follow-up studies involved parts of previously studied groups. Acheson noted "*It seems reasonable to suspect that a bias was operating in favour of patients with confirmed symptoms.*" But this contrasted with the follow-up studies in the Alaskan and

Punta Gorda outbreaks where all those in the original groups were involved. However, the Punta Gorda follow-up took place five months after the onset, whereas the Alaskan study was a two-year follow-up. At five months, only one patient in the Punta Gorda group was completely well, and the overall tendency was for a slow improvement with a fluctuating course. While more than half of the thirty patients were confined to bed at two months, in the sixth month only three were still bedridden. Many remained symptomatic: twelve suffered from depression; fifteen reported fatigue as a problem; eighteen noted nervous tension.

While all of the one hundred seventy-five patients in the Alaskan epidemic were re-assessed two years after the onset of their illness, the resulting data are incomplete, as there was no information about those who had improved, were well and had returned to work. Instead it was reported that of the one hundred seventy-five patients, one hundred and ten tired easily; eighty-one suffered from pain and stiffness; fifty-seven reported muscle weakness and sixteen were described as having "muscle paralysis." Even after two years, mental symptoms, which included emotional instability, poor concentration and memory defects, were extremely common.

In a "Summary of the clinical features," Acheson made the following observations:

(1) That there was a great deal of variability in the severity and/or the duration of any prodromal illness.

(2) Early symptoms included headache and pain in the neck, back and limbs, with little relationship to the presence or absence of fever.

(3) Muscular pain, headache and neck pain, were worst in the Los Angeles, Middlesex and Royal Free Hospital outbreaks, where the myalgia was described as "agonising" requiring narcotics for relief while varying in site and intensity from day to day.

(4) While upper body pain was present in some outbreaks, in others there was discomfort rather than pain.

(5) Numbness and tingling were common features in most cases.

(6) Urine retention, often requiring catheterisation, was recorded in eight outbreaks.

(7) Central nervous system involvement such as auditory disturbances showed considerable variation, but in all outbreaks emotional lability, lack of concentration and depression were reported frequently.

(8) In most cases, recovery was complete at one or two months, but in different outbreaks the journey to recovery was interrupted variably, by relapses.

Acheson concluded

In general, even in those patients (with neurological signs) there has been a trend to improvement, but in some instances a characteristic syndrome of chronic ill-health has developed, with cyclical recrudescences of pain, fatigue, weakness and depression, often coincident with menstruation, cold weather and exertion.

When writing about "Sporadic cases," Acheson drew attention to reports concerning small numbers of cases from widely disparate regions. While such cases showed many similar features and showed similarities to the events in the epidemic outbreaks, they occurred only in small numbers. By dismissing sporadic cases as being unimportant, Acheson was able to side-step the problem of explaining how the epidemic outbreaks were related to sporadic cases.

Acheson's observations concerning "Laboratory investigations," are summarised as follows:

(1) On the whole, the results from the examination of peripheral blood were unrewarding.
(2) In a few cases, ESR was raised.
(3) A positive Paul Bunnell test was extremely uncommon.
(4) Studies of cerebro-spinal fluid showed that normal cell counts were the rule, as were the protein levels, but an occasional lymphocytosis was noted.
(5) After electromyography of twenty eight patients from the Royal Free Hospital outbreak, Richardson noted that "…*the strength-duration curves were normal in all but one.*" However, Ramsay and Sullivan showed that on volition, motor unit potentials were grouped into sequences lasting from fifty to eighty milliseconds, and Galpine and Brady obtained similar results.

Those observations are in accord with the frequently expressed belief that in general, laboratory investigations are unrewarding, which draws attention to the lack of basic information about the nature of the disease process.

"Etiological studies" is the title of a section devoted to attempts to isolate etiologic agents. As shown in a large table, in many cases there were no virological investigations, and in nine of fourteen outbreaks there was no evidence of poliomyelitis or Coxsackie viruses. In the Bethesda outbreak, there was suggestive evidence of infection with "*…two strains of the Bethesda-Ballerup paracolon group*" in the faeces of twelve of thirty-eight nurses. It was noted "*It is possible that an unknown causative organism was being spread in addition to the Bethesda-Ballerup organism*" but as it involved less than a third of cases it is unlikely that the paracolon infection was a part of the epidemic disorder. No paracolon organisms were isolated from patients in the Punta Gorda group. A search for a possible "occupational toxic hazard" was unsuccessful. A possible role for insecticides, paints and detergents was sought during the Royal Free Hospital outbreak: the results were negative, as was the case in similar studies done in Bethesda and in Durban.

Thus there were no positive results from a number of searches for an etiologic agent. But it needs to be emphasised that even if it was possible to identify the presence of an agent, there remained a significant hurdle to be overcome to show how the agent was causally involved in the problem. The failure to identify a causal agent draws attention to the various reports of relapses being caused by energetic activity, cold weather and the onset of menstruation, which raises the question of how such disparate factors are involved.

In a chapter titled, "The case for a clinical entity," Acheson considered several possibilities:

(1) There was no evidence to support a proposal that poliomyelitis was involved.

(2) In considering a role for other enteric viruses, it was noted that in the reported outbreaks there was nothing which resembled the effects of Coxsackie or Echo viruses.

(3) The general pattern of the disorders did not fit that of encephalitis lethargica.

(4) Neither the nature of the disorder, nor the environmental requirements for arthropod-borne encephalitides were features of the outbreaks discussed.

(5) Infectious mononucleosis was seriously considered during the Royal Free Hospital outbreak, but was considered to be an unlikely agent.

(6) While other infectious agents were considered, none met the requirements.

So, at the completion of a search for a clinical entity, nothing suitable was found.

While considering the claims for the involvement of hysteria, Acheson noted that most authors considered that it had not contributed greatly to the pattern of the illness. Mental symptoms, which were an almost constant feature of all outbreaks, were incompatible with hysteria. This conclusion was reinforced by the mental dysfunction which was a common feature of convalescence. He concluded that

> *Final points against mass hysteria as a major factor in the syndrome are the consistency and course of the illness and the similarities in the symptoms described in spite of a wide variation in the types of community affected, from hospital staff on the one hand to semi-rural and urban populations on the other.*

Ramsay was much more direct and wrote as follows:

> *I consider the McEvedy and Beard hypothesis (that the Royal Free Hospital outbreak was due to mass hysteria) to be totally untenable and it is a matter for regret that it was ever put forward, nor can one explain why it was accepted so readily by the profession as a whole.*

In my later section I point out that the typical ME patient, with wide-ranging and variable symptoms, about which the doctor has been given conflicting advice, and for which there is no straightforward diagnostic procedure or treatment, presents a huge challenge. A challenge such as this may cause a doctor to wish, whole-heartedly, to be able to dismiss, perhaps even blame, the patient for their symptoms. This may provide some explanation of why 'the McEvedy and Beard hypothesis ... was accepted so readily by the profession as a whole'.

In a section titled, "The homogeneity of the material" Acheson compared and contrasted the situations in the different outbreaks. He pointed out that in fourteen of the outbreaks there was no evidence to show that any known neurotropic infection was involved. He also ruled out the possibility that the syndrome was "...*a self-perpetuating medical artefact.*" There were many differences in the findings related to the various outbreaks and in the lengths of the illness. He wrote

> *In its epidemic form, the illness is distinctive and therefore has a rightful place in the medical literature as a clinical entity. Its epidemiological features suggest it may be an infection. However, in the absence of any pathological evidence, it*

remains uncertain whether it is due to a single agent or to a group of related agents.

He recognised that for sporadic cases, a diagnosis required that the cases showed most of the features observed in epidemic outbreaks, together with a lack of evidence of viral involvement. However, he did not discuss what factor or factors could transform sporadic cases into an epidemic outbreak. Ramsay, on the other hand, considered that the sporadic cases in North West London between 1955 and 1958 could have been "*a nidus of infection*," with regard to the Royal Free Hospital epidemic.

Acheson recorded that there was no known treatment which affected the course of the disease, and emphasised the importance of rest. In addition he noted that it could be important to maintain bed rest for some time after the disappearance of symptoms, as had been suggested by others. This was considered to be necessary as "*The association of premature rehabilitation with relapse is well described.*"

As far as "Nomenclature" is concerned, Acheson wrote "The wisdom of naming a disorder, the nature of which cannot be proved, and which may be due to more than one agent, is debateable." Later he stated

In our present state of ignorance, 'encephalomyelitis' seems preferable to 'encephalopathy' because it conveys the suggestion that the disease in infective in origin, which is most certainly the case.

He concluded "It is unlikely that an adequate term will be found until fresh evidence is available."

In summarising his article, Acheson made the following points:

(1) Certain outbreaks of a paralytic illness of worldwide distribution are described.
(2) In twelve of those outbreaks, there were many similar features which could indicate either a single or a related group of causative agents.
(3) There was an unexplained preference for residential communities, with a higher attack rate in young adults, particularly in females.
(4) Outbreaks usually occurred in summer, with the possible spread by personal contact.
(5) Convalescence is usually prolonged; is associated with recurring fatigue and myalgia, and recovery is usually complete by three months.
(6) A proportion of cases will develop chronic ill health, with partial remissions and exacerbations marked by depression, emotional lability and a lack of concentration.
(7) Clinical laboratory studies have not been helpful.
(8) "No deaths directly attributable to the disease have occurred and the pathology remains unknown."
(9) No known viral or bacterial pathogen has been shown to be a causal agent.

In addition, the author wrote

It is concluded that the disease is recognisable in its epidemic form on clinical and epidemiological grounds and may therefore be considered a clinical entity. In its sporadic form, which is now well documented, the diagnosis should be reserved at present for severe cases with definite neurological signs, including paresis, and the characteristic fluctuating course. The disease is probably due to infection by an unknown agent or a group of related agents.

What is missing from the summary and conclusions is an explanation for why muscle and nerve tissue is most adversely affected, and why symptoms in such tissues are exacerbated by such unrelated phenomena as energetic activity, cold weather and the onset of menstruation. Is it possible that the rather small proportions of all cases which developed "chronic ill health" were cases of ME?

With regard to the worldwide distribution of the disorder, it is of interest that in 1982 there was an outbreak of an unexplained illness in Tapanui, a small country town in New Zealand, which gave rise to the term 'Tapanui 'flu.' Much of what was recorded about the illness resembles the epidemic outbreaks discussed by Acheson. Most cases developed in the spring and summer. Equal numbers of males and females made up the twenty-eight cases, and children under fifteen years of age comprised 35% of the group. Laboratory investigations of blood samples and searches for parasites produced no useful information. It was recorded that the disease had an acute phase of about five days which led into a chronic phase. Six patients had recovered in about five months but most of the patients were still experiencing symptoms about a year later. Of these, 40% had been symptomatic for more than five months. After becoming tired or stressed, some patients suffered a relapse. The symptom patterns but without the mental symptoms, were similar to those reported in other outbreaks. Sixteen cases reported that other members of their family had had a similar illness in the past.

Although many possible causes were investigated, none produced helpful information. The authors of the report could find no justification for calling the disease ME, and it became known as 'Tapanui flu'. An interesting aftermath was that after the publication of the report in June 1984, there were many reports of sporadic cases from different parts of New Zealand, many of which were diagnosed as ME.

So, what is the relevance of the epidemic outbreaks which occurred over more than forty years in the Pre-ME era, to ME? Perhaps the best interpretation would be to propose that the manifestations of the illness followed a post-infective stimulus, and in most cases the illness was of short duration. However, the minority, who suffered from moderate- to long-term, remitting/relapsing illness would be candidates for a diagnosis of ME. What this implies is that individuals in the ME group are in some way different to the majority, maybe in anatomy, physiology or in their immunological responses, and furthermore, that the difference is greater in females. It seems necessary to recognise that some difference exists in order to explain why relapses are triggered by such apparently unrelated factors as exertion, cold weather or the onset of menstruation.

The M.E. Era.

What follows is a selection of published comments, mainly in chronological order, which demonstrate the various shifts in opinion concerning the nature of ME, and the extent to which the concept of ME has met with resistance from much of the medical profession. To

85

a major degree, the acceptance of ME was greatly hindered by the 1988 release of the guidelines for chronic fatigue syndrome.

As a result of the suggestion in a Lancet editorial in 1956 (1) that the various outbreaks of chronic illness should be known as "benign myalgic encephalomyelitis" there was a retrospective naming of outbreaks before that date. However, although the name was adopted widely, there was criticism of the term "benign", which had been chosen because the illness had not been associated with deaths; and several authors had emphasised that the disorder itself was far from benign. However, between October 1956 and January 3, 1981 there were at least twenty-nine publications concerning 'benign myalgic encephalomyelitis'. International interest in the topic was reflected in publications in Switzerland, Israel, Greece, India and Lebanon.

In 1957 the British Medical Journal published an editorial titled, "Epidemic myalgic encephalomyelitis" (2) in the same issue as the report on the Royal Free Hospital outbreak, noting that there had been a number of outbreaks in different parts of the world in which encephalitis was a prominent feature. It was stated *"From published reports it is clear that no clue to the cause has yet been obtained, so that any assumption that such outbreaks are of the same aetiology is purely hypothetical."* But because of the recognisable similarities in clinical and epidemiological patterns *"... it seems justifiable to consider them as a medical entity."*

In the report on the Royal Free Hospital outbreak, it was stated that "Extensive investigations, with the help of outside laboratories have failed so far, to reveal either an infective agent or a causative factor." (3). The Royal Free report provided information about the manifestations, signs and symptoms of those involved. Headache, sore throat and malaise were the most frequent early symptoms, which changed variably in the second and third week when patients became more severely ill. Temperatures rarely exceeded 100 degrees F. Sometimes the illness involved the intensification of existing symptoms or new symptoms developed, such as sleep problems with nightmares, panic states or inexplicable, uncontrollable weeping. In addition, some cases developed vision problems, amnesia or limb pain. The report stated

> *The clinical impression was that this disease produced a diffuse disorder of the nervous system with a combination of irritative and paralytic signs, which were frequently transient.*

It was noted also that *"The course of the disease has been most variable."* Although symptoms and fever could abate for two or three weeks, such remissions were followed by relapses involving the old symptoms and sometimes with the appearance of new symptoms. Such changes led to anxiety and depression. **In the management of the acute phase, absolute rest provided the best outcome**, but convalescence was slow and was based upon the same length of time spent in the ward. Warm baths provided relief during physiotherapy exercises.

Laboratory investigations failed to produce useful information, although it was noted

The explosive character of the outbreak suggested the possibility that the infective agent was disseminated through a common vehicle, but investigations relating to water, milk, food, food-handlers and launderers were negative.

It was concluded, "In the absence of pathological evidence any view regarding the nature of the lesion in the Royal Free Hospital epidemic must remain hypothetical."

A paper titled, "Myalgic encephalomyelitis" published in 1961 (4) concerned two patients with case histories resembling the pattern reported in the Royal Free Hospital and Durban outbreaks. Although it was recognised that the illness was usually epidemic, the author stated, "*This illness is probably commoner than is usually realised, and mild, sporadic cases may easily be labelled as hysteria, glandular fever or myalgia.*"

While this observation was eventually shown to be true, progress to a better understanding of myalgic encephalomyelitis was halted temporarily by a claim in 1970 (5) that the Royal Free Hospital outbreak was a "hysterical phenomenon." In an accompanying paper (6), which reinforced the original proposal, the authors stated

We believe that these epidemics were psychosocial phenomena caused by one of two mechanisms, either mass hysteria on the part of the patients, or altered medical perceptions of the community.

They concluded

As there seems to be a total lack of support of the view that in cases of benign myalgic encephalomyelitis, the brain and spinal cord are the site of an infective, inflammatory disease, we would suggest the name be discarded......Our own inclination is for 'myalgia nervosa' on the analogy of anorexia nervosa.

This is the Beard and McEvedy report, based on the records of the ninety-two patients whom Dr. Ramsay had **already** excluded from his report, as he felt that they did not fit the ME pattern of symptomology. As a result of this, the medical profession were given information which **only** applied to people who Dr. Ramsay believed did **not** have ME: information according to which ME had been shown to be a form of 'mass hysteria'. This line of thinking about ME is alive and well, thanks to the Wessely group, with the term 'somatoform' replacing the term 'mass hysteria.'

In the same year, there was a report concerning four cases of encephalomyelitis which resembled benign myalgic encephalomyelitis (7). In three cases there was evidence of Coxsackie B virus infections, while echovirus type 3 was shown to be present in the fourth case. The author made two interesting observations:

Either we accept that different viruses can produce the same clinical picture, or we must seek some other explanation. It could be that all were affected by a common virus, the enteroviral infection being fortuitous.

Later he wrote

Could it be that enteroviral infection, in predisposed or previously sensitised subjects sets in train some process, say of an allergic nature, which accounts for the similarity of symptoms and the chronic relapsing course?

The author continued

> *We do not know if the chronic relapsing course in any way reflects lingering infection, or if the 'allergic' process is entirely self-perpetuating, or if severe relapses (and these occur, even after months of relative good health) are the result of re-exposure to the original virus or to a related virus.*

It is noteworthy that the author appeared to be unaware of the many observations which considered that relapses could be triggered by over-energetic activity, or cold weather or the onset of menstruation.

In an interesting comment on that paper, Lyle (8) referred to a simple writing test which might provide a measure of the rate of fatiguing. After the arm circulation was stopped by a sphygmomanometer cuff, the time the subject could continue to write was recorded. While a healthy subject stopped after 30 seconds *"The patient I asked to perform this test had to stop at 17 seconds. He gradually produced better times over the succeeding weeks."* However, the result was believed to imply *"a lesion distal to the cuff"* and a problem of blood flow was not considered. So as early as May 1970, it was shown that the flow properties of blood in an ME patient were in some way different, but the observation was before its time.

As part of a letter relating to the McEvedy and Beard hypothesis of hysteria, Parish (9) pointed out that two dangers arose from acceptance of that hypothesis. The greater danger would be the possible abandonment of the search for an understanding of the aetiology of the disorder. Secondly, he noted that *"...the patient may be labelled an hysteric and denied the assistance he would get if it was considered he had an organic disability."*

In a letter to Lancet, Ramsay et al (10) summarised the general features of Icelandic Disease/Royal Free Disease, and made a plea for sufferers who were still disabled to get in touch with a newly formed research group.

During the ensuing five years there was no apparent progress in understanding the events which led to myalgic encephalo-myelitis. An editorial in the British Medical Journal in 1978 (11) titled, "Epidemic myalgic encephalomyelitis" noted that *"We still know nothing about the nature and cause of epidemic myalgic encephalomyelitis."*

Behan (12) examined the possibility that acute disseminated encephalomyelitis and epidemic myalgic encephalomyelitis might share a common pathogenesis. Late in that paper, he stated that experimental allergic encephalitis (EAE) was regarded as the animal model of acute disseminated encephalomyelitis.

It is sheer coincidence that in the early 1990's I received blinded blood samples from a group in Sofia, Bulgaria, who were studying rats sensitised with myelin basic protein as a model of EAE. The immediately-fixed blood samples had been collected at different time intervals after the injection of the myelin basic protein. After the usual procedures and scanning electron microscopy, the micrographs were subjected to red cell shape analysis. The results were sent to Sofia, and the samples were identified. The results showed a steady, time-related increase in cells with altered margins (echinocytes) which was maximal just before death. Unfortunately, the group disbanded when the leader migrated to Australia and no further samples of EAE have been assessed.

But if, as Behan has suggested, there might be a common pathogenesis for both acute disseminated encephalomyelitis and epidemic myalgic encephalomyelitis, then maybe, as found in EAE, the primary problem could be changed shape populations of red cells which would impair capillary blood flow. Such a possibility would be consistent with the implications of the writing exercise reported by Lyle (8). So it is worth noting that in1989 I reported similar findings from blood samples from ME people.

Under the title, "Myalgic encephalomyelitis 'An obscene cosmic joke,'" the Medical Journal of Australia published a patient's viewpoint (13). After providing a description of her experience with the illness, the author expressed the view that it should be a notifiable disorder and stated *"The three common indicators are weakness, depression, and the pattern of relapse and recovery."* The author quoted Sir McFarlane Burnett

> *When a condition seems to have no obvious cause, it tends to be placed provisionally in the currently popular pigeon hole. It is probably only a slight exaggeration to say that over the past fifty years such conditions have been ascribed in sequence to, 'sceptic foci,' 'psychosomatic processes,' 'autoimmunity,' and now, 'slow viruses'*

This is a concept which is clearly relevant to the ME situation. Later she wrote

> *From the viewpoint of medicine functioning as a 'science' the concept of psychosomatic illness is marvellously convenient. It means that anything difficult to diagnose can be dismissed as not falling into a category needing assistance from medicine and patients can be handed over to psychiatrists to work out their 'failings'.*

Writing in a section called, "Brush up your medicine," Bishop (14) commented on epidemic myalgic encephalomyelitis, reiterating most of the observations reported by others. However, she noted

> *Relapses tend to be precipitated by too much physical activity (physiotherapy may produce a relapse), climatic changes, emotional tension, and from the writer's observations, inter-current viral infections or contact with viral infections in the patient's family.*

Rather surprisingly, the role of the onset of menstruation as a trigger for relapse, which had been reported by others was not mentioned, nor was there any discussion of how such diverse factors could lead to a relapse. Although it was stated, *"Both sexes and all age groups are affected. In many community outbreaks the sex incidence was equal"* but in fact this was the case in only three outbreaks (Adelaide, Dalston, Tapanui).

Church (15) drew attention to work by Ramsay and Rundle which showed that the results from biochemical tests of ME sufferers *"…were similar to those found in Duchenne Muscular dystrophy (DMD) though there are some important differences."*

It could be relevant that in the early 1970s there were several reports concerning red cell shape in muscular dystrophy patients. Only two of those studies examined immediately fixed blood samples, and one of these (16) reported that they were unable to prevent unfixed red cells from changing shape, even in their own plasma in the refrigerator.

A 1977 report showed that Huntington's Disease patients had high numbers of cup forms (stomatocytes), an observation which stimulates the question, "What common factor might be responsible for the changed red cell shape populations reported in experimental allergic encephalitis, muscular dystrophy and Huntington's Disease, and how does that factor relate to myalgic encephalomyelitis?"

An outbreak of benign myalgic encephalomyelitis in a girls' school in 1980 (17) in which the most frequent symptoms were headache, stomach ache, feeling sick and tiredness or weakness, led to the conclusion that a psychogenic factor was involved. It was concluded, *"The three broad conclusions of the international symposium – that the condition was a specific disease entity of viral and not psychogenic origin – were thus not substantiated."* The authors suggested that in future outbreaks, evidence should be sought for the involvement of both viral and psychogenic factors.

The findings in that paper were challenged by Goodwin (18) who considered the disease described in the paper, *"...is barely recognisable as myalgic encephalomyelitis,"* and gave reasons for holding that view. May et al (19) responded to this comment by stressing the belief that they were, *"...describing the same phenomenon as Ramsay and others."*

In September 1984, a consultant rheumatologist in Auckland, New Zealand, Dr. P. Gow (20) stimulated a flow of letters to the editor of the New Zealand Medical Journal when he suggested that current interest in ME in New Zealand resulted from, *"...media-directed attention to the ubiquitous occurrence of the somatic manifestations of stress, albeit triggered in many instances by a viral illness."* Dr. P. Snow (21) replied in the following month, pointing out that the decision to invite media interest was in keeping with fact that ME is a health problem and, *"...it is now recognised that the problem is a NZ-wide phenomenon and indeed a worldwide one."*

Simpson et al (22) stated that Dr. Gow's letter on ME *"... exemplifies current medical attitudes to those who suffer from a disorder of currently unexplained aetiology."* The idea that ME sufferers were waiting for a "magic bullet cure," conveyed no hint of sympathy for sufferers. In addition it was stated that work in progress showed that ME people had altered blood rheology, which was potentially treatable. It was concluded that, *"...those in the community who suffer from ME can be comforted by the fact that there is an organic cause for their illness and that it is not all in the mind."*

Dr. Gow replied on December 12, 1984 (23) writing critically about *"...diagnostic blood rheology as well as unsubstantiated therapeutic claims for nutrition quackery and Efamol etc.,"* showing very clearly that he was unfamiliar with the implications of altered blood rheology and how the effects might be alleviated. However, he did accept that stress, *"...including exercise stress will aggravate the fatigue state of patients with reduced endurance capacity,"* but he did not spell out how this occurred nor did he appear to understand that stress influenced blood rheology.

Dr. Gow's writings stimulated responses from others. Matthew (24) wrote, "I am concerned about the statements of Dr. Gow in your Journal and elsewhere, in relation to the aetiology and treatment of myalgic encephalomyelitis. It has already been pointed out that the notion of a psychogenic aetiology is against the consensus of medical opinion." He concluded, "I am grateful to those few doctors who are now familiar with myalgic encephalomyelitis and are providing support to families such as my own, by making the diagnosis, where appropriate."

Simpson et al (25) replied to Dr. Gow's comments relating to the role of blood rheology, stating that a paper had been submitted, but it was rejected by the British Medical Journal and eventually was published in Pathology (in 1986). In his reply (26) Dr. Gow gave the impression that he was well versed in haemorheology, but the correspondence was terminated by a contribution from Professor J.C. Murdoch (27) which stated, "...which brings us to the hub of the matter, with respect to Dr. Gow's research, presumably, '...properly controlled trials based upon testable hypotheses.' Both myalgic encephalomyelitis sufferers and researchers are waiting all agog to read the results of Dr. Gow's research." The letter concluded "Surely, if his position was clear in August 1984 he should now be in a position to reveal his hand and put us all out of our misery." A recent search of the literature failed to reveal any relevant publication by Dr. Gow. What this exchange of letters shows very clearly is the way in which the opinions of medically qualified writers provide obstacles to obtaining recognition of the problems of those with ME.

A hypothesis proposing a biochemical basis for myalgic encephalomyelitis was put forward in 1985 by Staines (28). It was stated, "The hypothesis is, therefore, that disruption of glycolysis in nerve and muscle tissue may occur through inactivation or inhibition of adenylate deaminase function. Moreover, such disruption may be a consequence of specific viral assault – for example by Coxsackie B infection. Such biochemical disruption could conceivably result in a syndrome consistent with that of myalgic encephalomyelitis."

But in many cases of myalgic encephalomyelitis it is not possible to demonstrate the presence of any virus, and if such a biochemical mechanism was involved it is difficult to understand how remissions which may last for hours, days or weeks might occur. And if adenylate deaminase was the crucial factor, it would need to be explained why such widely different stimuli as cold weather, physical activity and the onset of menstruation are triggers for relapses.

The publication of our paper in 1986 (29) which showed that ME blood filtered poorly in comparison with that of blood donor blood, provided a basis for considering that a primary factor in the development of ME was impaired capillary blood flow. This would lead to tissue dysfunction because of inadequate rates of delivery of oxygen and nutrient substrates.

In addition the paper stimulated an Australian group to study the red cells of ME patients after a relapse (30) which was published as a letter in Lancet in 1987. But as the cells were manipulated and centrifuged prior to fixation the study was compromised from the outset. It was reported that "Erythrocytes with normal morphology were rare," and attention was focussed upon "dimpled spherocytes." However, as I have never seen such cells in more than 13,000 immediately fixed blood samples, it is likely that they are artefacts of preparation.

The authors of the study agreed with our proposal that poorly deformable red cells could impair blood flow in the microcirculation. Although they quoted a study which showed changed red cell shape populations in athletes who had completed a marathon, their literature search was incomplete, as between April 1974 and January 1983 there were four published reports concerning red cell shape in muscular dystrophy. But only two studies used immediately fixed red cells (16, 31) and they reported increased cup forms (stomatocytes) while the reports relating to samples which had been manipulated prior to fixation showed increased cells with altered margins (echinocytes).

In addition, Markesbery and Butterfield (32) in 1977 reported that increased numbers of stomatocytes were present in the blood of patients with Huntington's Disease, and in 1984 Yasuda et al (33) reported that in immediately fixed blood samples from cases of spinocerebellar degeneration there were increased numbers of echinocytes. Furthermore, they noted that, *"The procedures before fixation greatly affect the shape of erythrocytes."* So although there is a body of information which links different pathological conditions to changed shape populations of red cells, a key factor is the immediate fixation of the blood samples.

This point is really important – "a key factor is the immediate fixation of the blood samples." If blood samples are not immediately fixed, the red blood cells revert to the supposedly typical biconcave discocyte form, and the evidence supporting Dr. Simpson's information – that predominance of shape-changed, inflexible blood cells in ME results in oxygen deprivation in areas dependent upon small capillaries and this produces the symptoms of ME – is lost.

Such observations increase the possibility that the unusual results published by Mukherjee et al (30) were artefacts of preparation. Change in the shape populations of red cells has its physiological consequences and Pantely et al (34) showed that shape-transformed red cells reduced the rate of capillary blood flow velocity, while Kon et al (35) reported that a reduction in the rate of capillary blood flow reduced the rate of erythrocyte de-oxygenation. In an in vitro study, Vandergriff and Olson (36) showed that both the uptake and release of oxygen was reduced in echinocyte-transformed red cells. Those papers provide access to an interesting literature. As shape change is associated with a reduction in deformability (as shown by filterability) (29), it is clear that change in the shape populations of red cells is not a benign event, yet there is no current recognition of its pathological potential.

Of the two hundred cases of ME which Murdoch described in 1987 (37), the majority had been ill since 1983. He stated "The clinical findings strongly suggest that the musculature and central nervous system are the main sites of disorder in these patients." Such an observation draws attention to the fact that both types of tissue – muscle and nerve cells – are particularly sensitive to oxygen deprivation and would be at risk when there were changes in the shape populations of red cells, or when red cells became poorly deformable as noted previously (34, 35). Although a wide range of laboratory tests were carried out, in none of the tests was there a majority with abnormal results. Therefore it was important that Murdoch should conclude that "The patients with recognisable abnormalities were no more or less sick than those without."

For ME sufferers, the year 1988 was marked by a number of important events, such as the publication of the second edition of Ramsay's book, and in the Preface he emphasised the "*clear distinction*" between ME and the post-viral fatigue (PVFS) states. He wrote "*The wrongful assumption that ME and PVFS are synonymous, now prevalent in the world literature on the subject, serves to blur the true clinical identity of the myalgic encephalomyelitis syndrome.*"

On p 24 it was noted that during the Finchley outbreak in 1964-66, "A diagnosis of ME was never considered unless most of the following features were present: low grade fever and headache, blurred vision and/or diplopia, stiff neck, vertigo with a positive Romberg test, nausea and/or vomiting, lymphadenopathy, lower costal or generalised muscular weakness unrelieved by rest, emotional lability, insomnia and/or vivid dreams, often in colour, frequency or retention of urine, varying degrees of deafness or hyperacusis."

But when he considered the endemic form of the illness this was discussed under three headings, namely, muscle phenomena, circulatory impairment and cerebral dysfunction. Possibly due to hindsight, it is strange that he did not consider that circulatory impairment might be involved in the muscular and cerebral dysfunction.

However, when considering the papers which follow, it is important to keep in mind Ramsay's cardinal features of ME; the unique form of muscle fatigability with a lengthy time lapse before the restoration of muscle power; the variability of symptoms and physical signs during a day; and the tendency toward chronicity. In addition it could be rewarding to think about how impaired capillary blood flow might contribute to the tissue dysfunction manifested as symptoms.

And 1988 saw the introduction of Chronic Fatigue Syndrome, with its consequent confusion. While the topic will be considered in the "Post-ME Era," it appears frequently in the ME literature. As an example, the appropriateness of the term myalgic encephalomyelitis was considered in 1988 (38). It was concluded that the terms myalgic encephalomyelitis and post-viral fatigue syndrome were inappropriate and it was suggested that the disorder be named "*idiopathic chronic fatigue and myalgia syndrome.*" But in the discussion concerning aetiology, the matter of remissions was not addressed, nor was there any role assigned to impaired blood flow.

In replying to a critical letter, the author, Byrne, (39) commented on the findings of Mukherjee et al (30) and stated, "*...it is not immediately clear what their significance might be in the pathoetiology of this fatiguing condition.*" He claimed "*...the name myalgic encephalomyelitis was derived, essentially, from the observation of non-organic neurological symptomatology,*" when in fact, it was adopted because, according to Acheson, it implied an infective process.

Bell et al (40) reported that in two hundred and forty-seven patients admitted to a psychiatric hospital, 12.5% had significantly raised antibody titres to Coxsackie B virus. When sera from two hundred and ninety ME patients were tested by a new ELISA test 37% were positive to Coxsackie B virus IgM, which contrasted with 9% positivity in five hundred healthy adult controls. Although this showed that both healthy and unwell patients may be positive to tests for Coxsackie B virus, as far as ME is concerned, the relevance is dubious as the majority were negative.

LESLIE O. SIMPSON & NANCY BLAKE

A letter by an Australian group (41) published in Lancet under the title, "What is myalgic encephalomyelitis ?" stimulated a controversy as the letter seemed to explain the reasons for the adoption of the CDC concept of chronic fatigue syndrome. In fact the letter might have been titled better, "What is chronic fatigue syndrome?"

The letter provoked critical comments from Drs Ramsay and Dowsett and praise from the staff of the Institute of Psychiatry. Dr. Ramsay rejected the claim that the term myalgic encephalomyelitis was inappropriate. He stated that post-infectious states "...*are clinically in complete contrast to the three cardinal features of ME – namely, a unique form of muscle fatigability, whereby, even after a minor degree of physical effort, three or more days elapse before full muscle power is restored; the extraordinary variability or fluctuation of symptoms even in the course of one day; and the alarming chronicity which exceeds anything encountered in a post-viral fatigue state."* (42)

Writing in similar vein, Dr. Dowsett (43) stated, "The introduction of 'chronic fatigue syndrome' to designate ME does nothing to indicate the unique epidemiological, geographical, clinical and laboratory findings in ME and can only add to the confusion surrounding the diagnosis, therapy and prognosis of the condition."

David et al (44) commended the authors for considering the case definition of chronic fatigue syndrome, and noted, "Clinical descriptions stress emotional lability and severe depression, so that psychological disturbance seems central to the disorder." In addition they stated "The greatest challenge facing researchers will be to distinguish fatigue as a symptom of depressive illness, depression as a consequence of chronic fatigue and depression as an integral part of a new disease entity."

> As an experienced psychotherapist who also has personal experience of ME, I would point out two things, which I have mentioned elsewhere:
>
> 1) Having a relatively sudden onset of a seriously disabling condition for no apparent reason is an extremely emotionally upsetting experience. It would be abnormal not to be emotionally upset by this.
>
> 2) The nature of the illness is that one has the same vulnerability to tearfulness as that which would be experienced by anyone in a state of extreme physical exhaustion. One can be experiencing this tearfulness when perfectly happy; it is not a sign of a psychiatric disorder or even of being particularly emotionally distressed.
>
> In response to the author's concern about how to 'distinguish fatigue as a symptom of depressive illness, depression as a consequence of chronic fatigue, and depression as an integral part of a new disease entity', the first distinction is extremely easy to make. The depressed person lacks motivation to do anything, but if pushed to get a little exercise, will find their mood lifted. The person with ME is motivated to do things, will attempt them, find they are unable to continue, and become very upset about this. If exercise makes you feel better, you have not got ME. If it makes you feel worse, the chances are that you do.

Of course anyone with a longer-term experience of ME will have learned that they pay a heavy price for over-exertion, and will therefore, justifiably, resist attempts to force them to go beyond their limits. Enthusiasts of the idea that ME is a 'somatoform disorder' will interpret this very realistic behaviour as further proof of their hypothesis.

But having shown that blood rheology is not normal in ME people (29), it seems reasonable to consider that both muscle fatigability and depression could be manifestations of impaired capillary blood flow, because, as noted previously, both muscle and nerve tissue are particularly sensitive to oxygen deprivation. It should be noted also that there are several studies relating to regional cerebral blood flow as observed by SPECT, in depressive illness, which show reduced rates of blood flow in various parts of the brain. One such study showed that during an episode of depression, there was a reduction in regional cerebral blood flow, but after the resolution of the depression, blood flow returned to normal in that region.

Late in 1988, Murdoch (45) reviewed the "Myalgic encephalomyelitis syndrome," and discussed the position in the United Kingdom, North America and New Zealand. He stated *"It would be important to know, for example, whether they are all describing the same phenomenon and whether this is similar to what has been described in the past as myalgic encephalomyelitis."* He continued *"It is unlikely that the relationship between the present phenomenon and all those outbreaks will ever be conclusively established"* but *"The search for an aetiology for this condition has been frustrating, since no one factor seems to be entirely responsible."*

In addition the author wrote

> *Recently it has been suggested that impaired microcirculation and altered blood rheology may account for the plethoric but relapsing symptomatology, and altered red cell morphology has been described.*

However, it is unlikely that the writer was aware that any event which changed the red cell environment, such as the immune responses to infections, stress or emotional upsets, and hormonal changes would stimulate changes in the shape populations of red cells and reduce red cell deformability. The consequences of poorly deformable red cells would be most severe in those randomly distributed regions which had a majority of small capillaries, implying that there would be a wide range of responses to similar changes in the shape populations of red cells. Furthermore, as the red cells would revert to normal when their environment was normalised, this could provide an understanding of the mechanism of remissions.

Murdoch concluded

> *The experience from New Zealand is that many otherwise well-trained physicians prefer not to deal with these profound but simple issues and, after a fruitless search for intellectual clues, leave the patient in the limbo of having '...nothing physically wrong,' where they have to choose between admitting madness or going to seek the help of complementary therapies. Being able to help such people challenges academic family medicine to its very core and in particular to produce the physicians who are equipped to take on this task.*

95

In 1989, Simpson (46) reported that scanning electron microscopy of immediately fixed blood samples from one hundred and two volunteers who believed that they suffered from ME, revealed that they had higher percentages of cup-transformed red cells (stomatocytes) and lower percentages of biconcave discocytes than healthy subjects. The expected effects of such cells would explain the poor filterability of ME blood reported in 1986 (29).

Later in the year the British Journal of Haematology published my paper which showed that the red blood cells of healthy animals and humans could be classified on the basis of simple criteria into six different shape classes.

Wessely (47) published a paper with the strange title, "Myalgic encephalomyelitis – a warning: discussion paper". This provided a good example of the confusion which followed on from the introduction of chronic fatigue syndrome. Despite the title, it is difficult to locate the warning, and the term ME was mentioned twice in the first seven lines and then is transformed into PVFS or CFS. As the majority of the text dealt with CFS, it is difficult to find anything which relates to the title of the paper. In the absence of any concept of cause or aetiology, it was not surprising that the author wrote

> It is this author's belief that patients seen in primary care with persistent fatigue shortly after an acute infection represent a very different population from those with longer periods of illness who are seen in hospital practices.

While such a viewpoint would seem to deny the findings from epidemic outbreaks, the nature of the warning remains obscure.

There were many responses to a topic "For debate," published in the British Medical Journal, titled, "Myalgic encephalomyelitis, Princess Aurora and the wandering womb," (48) which cast doubts about the relevance of ME. Although three critical comments were published, the editor noted that fourteen other letters had made similar points. Andrea Collingridge, from the ME Association stated that the article "…*would cause anger, distress and more distrust of doctors.*" She concluded "*Am I naïve in believing that we must all try to build trust and collaboration between patients and doctors to make this important task (patient management) easier?*"

Another correspondent, (L. Hartnell) stated

> What is even more intriguing is that an illness with the controversial label of myalgic encephalomyelitis, apparently suggests that every patient with that label – whether rightly or wrongly applied – is, in the words of the article, 'scenting a new career as patient.'"

The writer noted

> It seems totally incomprehensible that genuine patients should be ridiculed without a fair hearing because they have a certain medical label, albeit a little understood one or a controversial one.

This was followed by a question:

> What does the medical world feel that people gain by being disabled, cut off from society, hauled up before tribunals, suffering pain and discomfort?

and "Surely the sweeping attitude that patients enjoy being ill is itself sick."

96

In contrast, another correspondent (R.G. Walker) stated "Like Caroline Richmond I too feel that 'ME' is a medical fashion which I hope will die out as the others have."

Such correspondence, to a very great extent, shows clearly the great disparity in the ways in which society perceives myalgic encephalomyelitis as an illness.

In a critical commentary of the views which Dr. Charles Shepherd had expressed concerning muscle fatigue, Coakley (49) wrote as follows:

> *Patients with myalgic encephalomyelitis deserve a sympathetic approach from doctors, who should be prepared to believe their symptoms are genuine, whether they arise in mind or body. Advice should be given to enable them to cope with their symptoms, gradually increase their exercise tolerance and return to normality. Psychological support may be helpful. What is not needed is any further attempt to pursue the holy grail of the cause of muscle fatigue, because it does not exist.*

But this very definite opinion is at odds with the view of physiologists. In his 'Textbook of physiology', Griffiths (50) stated that muscle fatigue was due to oxygen deficiency, and the effects of localised accumulations of metabolites which were not removed when capillary blood flow was impaired. A similar opinion was expressed by Wiles et al (51) who considered muscle fatigue as the consequence of inadequate energy generation, the limiting factors for which were blood flow and oxygen delivery. Such viewpoints provide an explanation for the limiting effects of writing after vascular occlusion described by Lyle. (8) Because of the recognised effects of shape-changed red cells on the rate of oxygen delivery, it would seem very likely that when the shape populations of red cells are changed, they will contribute to the fatigability of muscles.

In July 1989, Murdoch reviewed the published information in an article titled "The myalgic encephalomyelitis syndrome." (52) He quoted Werry who suggested that during diagnostic probing, it

> *"...should be made clear to the patient for what it really is – our acceptance that something is wrong and that this is our fumbling for a diagnosis, not the assignment of one."*

At the conclusion of his review of relevant research he wrote

> *Fatigue, pain and emotional upset are the most common problems affecting humanity, and yet we understand little about their causation*

His final sentence stated "Much more research needs to be done on this difficult subject before any of us can have the privilege of being dogmatic."

Dr. Peter Snow (53) wrote

> *I wish to support Professor Campbell Murdoch's plea for an extensive research programme into the syndrome known as myalgic encephalomyelitis.*

While conceding that the costs of research would be high, he noted

> *I believe the normal difficulties of finding the funds will be compounded because of the apparent lack of acceptance of the syndrome from within the hierarchy of the*

medical profession, which makes the approval of funds from traditional funding sources almost impossible.

In addition it could be noted that the same lack of acceptance of the syndrome poses problems in having relevant studies published.

In reviewing ME from a South African perspective, Spracklen (54) equated ME with CFS and wrote

The chronic fatigue syndrome (CFS) or myalgic encephalomyelitis, has caused great confusion, misunderstanding and perhaps mismanagement of many persons presenting with a variety of combinations of ill-defined complaints.

When considering the pathogenesis of the problem, Spracklen made the significant observation that

The popular viral aetiology and the number of proposed pathogens raises the possibility that they may merely be NON-SPECIFIC, BIOLOGICAL OR PSYCHOBIOLOGICAL STRESSORS. (My emphasis)

Such a concept implies that the pathogens stimulate a common response such as stimulating change in the shape populations of red cells. In addition he stated

An undisputed feature of CFS is fatigue, and terms such as malaise, lassitude, tiredness, exhaustion, weakness and myalgia may complicate the issue. There is no question that fatigue is worsened by exercise, which may produce fatigue lasting for days or for several weeks. It is interesting that fatigue has been noted to follow both mental and physical effort. The possibility that psychological strain may induce disorders of muscle metabolism is interesting.

But in my experience ME people complain of tiredness rather than fatigue, and Sir John Ellis had written "*...although malaise and fatigue are terms which occur throughout medical textbooks, patients hardly ever use these terms.*" Although the dictionary definition of fatigue is *"to exhaust the strength by severe or long continued exertion"* in common usage fatigue appears to be equated with tiredness. However ME people do not have to exert themselves to invoke their pervasive tiredness.

As the effects of exercise are very relevant it is of some significance that regular, light exercise has been shown to reduce blood viscosity whereas heavy exercise increases blood viscosity and changes the shape populations of red cells and reduces their deformability.

Spracklen appeared to be much more impressed by the CDC definition of CFS, than by "*...Ramsay's simple triad of unique muscle fatigability, extraordinary variability of symptoms and alarming chronicity,*"

Although blood samples were obtained from ME people in several South African cities, the South African Medical Journal rejected the report containing the results obtained from the samples.

Writing about fatigue in ME, the late Martin Lev (of Action for ME) drew attention to the different responses to physical activity of those with depression and from those with ME (55). However, as patients with depression or with ME have been shown to have reduced regional cerebral blood flow (which could imply altered blood rheology) the responses to physical activity may not be clear cut. But Lev asked also, *"Might there not be some underlying organic processes going on which cause psychiatric symptoms?"* It is possible that the question is very relevant as it has been reported that SPECT scans of patients with different types of psychiatric disorder showed differences in regional cerebral blood flow, so the *"underlying organic process"* could be reduced cerebral blood flow.

The reactions of two general practitioners and a psychiatrist to a hypothetical case of self-diagnosed ME provided some insight into the reactions of physicians (56). Although a male general practitioner would do a full examination and order many blood tests, he stated *"I confess to a degree of scepticism about ME."* But he concluded *"Lastly, if other diagnoses are excluded, I will have made sure that I am now in a position to give an informed opinion about ME."* The second general practitioner was female, who stated *"I would assure Mary that ME is a relatively benign disease and is self-limiting"* It could be noteworthy that the doctor appears still to be influenced by the early name of benign myalgic encephalomyelitis. Because of her belief in underlying depression, after doing a number of blood tests, she would offer help through a psychologist. The psychiatrist, a male, was not impressed by the self-diagnosis and commented that ME is messy, difficult and controversial, and that ME is a description, not a diagnosis. *"If blood tests are normal, I would not investigate further."* If there is any good news for ME sufferers in this study, it is that the male general practitioner could be willing to make a diagnosis of ME on the basis of exclusion.

Prasher et al (57) reported a study in which ME patients had their brain stem, visual and somatosensory potentials measured. The ME group comprised twenty patients with positive responses to enteroviral antigen (VPI+) and twelve patients who were VPI negative. It was found that those who were VPI positive were not significantly different in terms of cognitive potential abnormalities from those who were VPI negative. Possibly the problems in selecting a "uniform" group for study could explain why some patients had attentional deficits and a slower speed of information processing than others. The authors wrote *"The sensory potentials of the visual, auditory, brainstem and median nerve somatosensory systems remain unaffected in ME."* However, given the evidence of altered blood rheology in ME people, it would be surprising if some aspects of brain function were not altered by impaired blood flow in the brain, which would relate to the random distribution of small capillaries.

Lynch and Seth (58) responded to Martin Lev's letter (55) concerning the nature of depression in ME people, emphasising the need to control for a range of variables. They noted, as many had done previously, that *"The concept of fatigue is poorly understood, as is its assessment."* In addition they stated *"…ME patients have more variability and unpredictable onset of fatigue relative to the severity of exercise attempted."* However, they did not address Lev's specific question concerning the possibility that some organic factor might cause psychiatric symptoms.

About nine months after the death of Dr. A. M. Ramsay, a paper by Dowsett, Ramsay et al (59) reported the results from an investigation into the possibility that myalgic encephalomyelitis might be the consequence of a persistent enteroviral infection.

Four hundred and twenty patients who met the criteria for ME were selected from six thousand cases with various infections, seen over a twelve year period. As 73% were female, the male:female ratio was 1:2.6. More than one-third, (37%) were aged between thirty-one and forty years and the male:female ratio for the age group was also 1:2.6.

A prodrome had occurred as a 'flu-like' illness with respiratory/gastrointestinal involvement, in 81% of patients, while 19% reported an insidious onset. Between 70% and 100% of patients reported muscle fatigue, emotional lability, myalgia, cognitive disturbance, headache and giddiness/disequilibrium.

The illness had persisted for from three to sixty years, and in 47% of cases, the illness had lasted from three to ten years while 12% had been ill for eleven to twenty years. A rather surprising feature was that only 20% had a fluctuating illness, which was a lower percentage than those reported to be improving, or who had a steady level of disability with no remissions. Such findings appear to be at odds with the selection criteria, which included, "*...a prolonged relapsing course.*"

But all participants relapsed after physical or mental stress. Other precipitants of relapses included surgery, immunization and hormonal disturbance. (It should be noted that all three factors have been shown to change the shape populations of red cells.)

While laboratory investigations showed some changes in minorities, the highest positive test (45%) concerned those with evidence of circulating immune antibodies. Such findings were similar to the 1987 findings of Murdoch (37). In the discussion, the possible mechanisms for a viral aetiology of ME were explored, but no explanation was provided for the fact that only a minority gave positive results. On the basis of the role of Coxsackie viruses, in the "*...deleterious effect of forced exercise on persistently infected muscles*" it was concluded that "*These studies elucidate the exercise-related morbidity and the chronic relapsing nature of ME.*" But such a claim ignores the fact that only a minority were positive for the presence of virus and it did not attempt to explain what happened during remissions. The authors concluded "*Clinical, laboratory and epidemiological data support the suggestion that ME is a complication of non-immune individuals of widespread, sub-clinical, non-polio-enterovirus infection.*" But such a conclusion cannot account for those cases of ME which followed exposure to herbicidal spray drift or a severe emotional upset.

An editorial titled "Myalgic encephalomyelitis: an alternative theory," by Wilson, (60) began with critical comments on an earlier paper by Wessely. He stated

> *It seems that a new kind of approach, based on the absence of prejudice, more exhaustive and thorough clinical history-taking, a wider approach to clinical examination of patients, and a critical assessment of the origin of this PSYCHOSOMATIC DISEASE (my emphasis) would be of value in our investigations.*

Evidently his previous experience (ten of sixteen quoted references concerned his own work) provided the basis for the claim that ME is a psychosomatic disease. It was stated

> *Three of the most important clinical diagnostic signs in ME patients are: the allergic family history which is invariably present, the seasonal and circadian rhythms of the somatic and mental symptoms in patients, and the fact that central*

nervous and psychiatric symptoms tend to persist after the somatic symptoms have begun to diminish.

It is noteworthy that no reference was made to any of the published reports concerning both epidemic and endemic ME, as none mention any *"…allergic family history"*. Furthermore it would be very difficult to interpret the occurrence of remissions and epidemic outbreaks in terms of chronic allergies, and this was not attempted. It was claimed that patients with persistent allergic disease may develop an Alternative Multiple Personality, a complicated situation that develops without the patient being aware of the change. The complex nature of this claim is exemplified by the statement that *"These psychopathological patients learn to reproduce allergic symptoms in the absence of any allergic antigen-antibody challenge."* As there is no attempt to relate his concept to the findings of others working in the field of ME, this editorial provides a good example of some of the extreme views which have been accepted into the literature. Such publications can only impede progress into gaining an understanding of ME.

Wessely (61) responded to Wilson's paper and wrote in rather cynical vein about some of the quoted references. For example, he stated

> *Similarly I would not have known that an article in the 'Christian Parapsychologist' called, 'Deliverance and dowsing,' is on the psychopathology of allergy and ME, nor that information on treatment of ME would be published in a series of titles beginning with 'Current theological perspectives on possession'.*

I am left with the impression that Dr. Wessely and I share similar views on Wilson's "Alternative theory on ME".

At the Cambridge Symposium on ME in April 1990, I presented my findings from the red cell shape analysis of a further ninety-nine cases of ME, (62) which were similar to those published in 1989 (46). In addition I reported the chance observation that people with acute ME (and increased cup forms) responded to injections of vitamin B12 as hydroxocobalamin by reducing symptom severity which was associated with lower numbers of cup-transformed red cells. For unexplained reasons, only 50% of cases responded.

During much of 1991 and 1992, a great deal of the material published involved ME as a synonym for CFS or for PVFS. Papers dealing with ME were published in nursing or other journals which were not available for review.

What should have been a major event for ME was the publication of the book titled, "The Clinical and Scientific Basis of Myalgic Encephalomyelitis/Chronic Fatigue Syndrome," edited by Drs. Hyde, Goldstein and Levine. Unfortunately for those who attended the Cambridge Symposium on Myalgic Encephalomyelitis, **there is no record of the proceedings of the symposium**, and that information has been lost to posterity. The "Foreword" of the book makes it clear that

> *This text that provides a basis of general information for clinicians and researchers interested in ME/CFS was initiated by the Cambridge Easter Symposium on Myalgic Encephalomyelitis/Chronic Fatigue Syndrome.*

It seems that it is irrelevant that it was the Cambridge Symposium on ME and it is not made clear how the symposium transformed into the ME/CFS symposium. As more than a third of the book is written by Americans about CFS, in papers which have little relevance to ME, from the viewpoint of ME sufferers, the book was a major disappointment. Even though Dr. Ramsay was honoured by being appointed "Honorary Chairman" of the symposium, his opinions were in general disregarded and were swamped by the sheer volume of American opinion relating to CFS.

In his presentation with Dr. Dowsett, Dr. Ramsay made three points concerning the aetiology, pathogenesis and prognosis of ME. He stated

> *First, there has been an absence of objective evidence of organic disease from laboratory and other studies, often leading to an inappropriate diagnosis of psychiatric or other behavioural disturbance. Second, the failure to distinguish the characteristic fatigue of myalgic encephalomyelitis from other, more short-lived post-infective disability (e.g. following influenza or infectious mononucleosis) or from other causes of fatigue, has led to unrealistic estimates of recovery. Third, the failure to agree on firm diagnostic criteria has distorted the data base for epidemiological and other research, thus denying the unique epidemiological pattern of myalgic encephalomyelitis.*

Subsequent to the publication of the book, its influence was soon manifested by the common usage of ME/CFS which simply served to confuse the diagnostic picture.

It is of some significance that the 1988 criteria for CFS had been the subject of critical comment for some years. A good example of this situation is a letter by Hume (63) of the ME Association in an exchange of opinions concerning the self-diagnosis of ME. Hume wrote

> *The main reason why our beliefs tend to differ from those of S. Wessely and H Cope and AS David, is that the authors do not distinguish between myalgic encephalomyelitis and chronic fatigue syndrome, as we do.*

In 1993 we published a paper titled "Red cell shape changes following trigger finger fatigue in subjects with chronic tiredness and healthy controls." (64) The title of the paper reflects the fact that the local ethics committee ruled that as ME was an undefinable disorder, the term ME was not permitted to be used in the title. Ethics committee approval was forthcoming when ME was replaced with, "subjects with chronic tiredness."

As it had been found that marathon runners had increased percentages of cup forms at the end of the marathon, and that exercycling by CFS patients was followed by a reduction in regional cerebral blood flow as assessed by SPECT, the study set out to explore the effects of inducing fatigue in a small muscle mass. This was achieved by repeatedly pulling a trigger until the onset of trigger finger fatigue. Most of the study was carried out at a weekend residential meeting of ME groups and controls were members of the police, fire service, army, teachers and nurses. After providing informed consent, participants provided a three drop sample of blood which was fixed immediately. The trigger was pulled until the onset of fatigue and a second blood sample was obtained. The elapsed time and the number of trigger pulls were recorded. Five minutes later the procedure was repeated. After the blood samples had fixed for overnight, at least, the blood cells were prepared for and photographed by scanning electron microscopy under standard conditions. The resulting micrographs were subjected to red cell shape analysis.

The results showed that the red cell shape populations of ME people in the pre-trigger pulling samples were significantly different from those of controls, as had been found in previous studies. ME people had fewer trigger pulls than healthy controls, the differences in the red cell shape populations had increased, and the differences were greater after the second series of trigger pulls. **The results from this simple study provide a basis for understanding the role of physical activity as a trigger for relapses, in terms of shape-changed, poorly deformable red cells**.

As it has been shown that many different agents, which alter the red cell environment, stimulate change in the shape populations of red cells, the findings enable the role of a large range of stressors which stimulate a relapse to be understood. Because the ethics committee would not approve a study which involved multiple blood samples from individuals, which would be needed to assess the time taken for exercise-induced changes in the shape populations of red cells to revert to the pre-exercise level, the time for reversion is not known.

As the numbers of blood samples from ME people continued to rise, in order to obtain some indication from general practitioners of the usefulness of the results of red cell shape analysis, an anonymous questionnaire was sent to the twenty-four general practitioners who had sent in blood samples in the period 1/7/93 to 31/12/93. All questionnaires were returned, and 78% of general practitioners considered the results were helpful or very helpful. While 96% of responders considered the results were useful for explanations to patients, 74% noted that the results influenced decisions on diagnosis and treatment. It was concluded that despite the small sample size, the general level of approval could indicate that a greater use of red cell shape analysis would result in a more logical approach to the management of patients with myalgic encephalomyelitis.

Another unpublished study set out to try and assess the frequency of remissions. A panel of thirty-seven women and eleven men, who had had a physician's diagnosis of ME more than two years previously and were chronically unwell, gave informed consent to participate. The group met every four weeks for forty weeks, to provide a blood sample, a list of symptoms and an estimate of well-being. The blood samples were subjected to standard procedures and the resulting scanning electron micrographs assessed by red cell shape analysis.

The results showed marked month-to-month variation which ranged from the experience of five women who had abnormal results for all eleven blood samples, to the woman who had six of eleven samples with normal values. Eleven women and three men had two samples with normal values while smaller numbers had three to five normal samples. While most samples had high values for flat cells there were a small number of samples with increased percentages of cells with altered margins or with surface changes, all of which are characteristic of chronic ME.

Although there was an occasional sample with increased cup forms (the marker for acute ME) they were probably the consequence of an inter-current infection, as they never persisted. An interesting finding was that participant's estimates of well-being correlated poorly with the results from red cell shape analysis. It seemed reasonable to conclude that because of the time period between sampling, the identification of remissions would be minimal, which suggests that remissions were not uncommon events.

However, as has been shown by others, the consequences of changed red cell shape populations with poorly deformable cells are reduced rates of delivery of oxygen and nutrient substrates. This becomes important in working muscle, which requires extra oxygen and substrates to produce the energy to do the work involved. If the metabolic needs of the working muscle are not met, there could be a switch to anaerobic respiration with a lower level of energy release, lactic acid formation and muscle pain, before the onset of muscle fatigue. While such a proposal would explain the easy fatigability of ME muscle, there is no available evidence which would confirm the variable time to recovery is related to the restoration of the pre-work shape populations of red cells.

Furthermore, reduced rates of delivery of the metabolic needs of tissues will impair endocrine gland and nerve tissue function, and are very likely to be involved in manifestations of brain dysfunction, such as memory problems and confusion.

There are direct parallels with the brain problems of ME and those of patients with Huntington's Disease, who like people with acute ME have increased cup forms (33). In 1985, Tanahashi et al (65) reported that by means of a Xenon washout technique they had found that Huntington's Disease patients had reduced rates of cerebral blood flow which correlated with the level of cognitive dysfunction. However, there was no reference to the changed red cell shape populations which had been reported eight years earlier, despite the fact that the increased cup forms were the probable cause of the observed reduction in blood flow.

With the objective of obtaining information about the status of patients with ME who had had red cell shape analysis between 1/7/92 and 31/12/95, a questionnaire containing seven questions was mailed to two hundred and twenty subjects randomly selected from nine hundred and twenty-six individuals. Replies were received from thirty-five males and ninety-two females (male to female ratio 1:2.6) and 14% considered that they were well while 49% (fifty-one cases) remained unwell. Those who became unwell at an early age had a shorter history of sickness and a better restoration of health. Thirty-nine (31%) were in full time employment and fifty (39%) were disabled. While a total of thirty-one different symptoms were listed, the four most worrisome symptoms were tiredness (22%), fatigue (21%), pain (8%) and memory problems (4%). Although 13% reported benefits from injections of vitamin B12 as hydroxocobalamin and 12% responded to evening primrose oil, the majority had failed to find a helpful treatment and remained unwell. As the costs of treatment could be a significant factor, it is not known if those who failed to benefit had had adequate treatment.

Because it is recognised that the average diameter of capillaries is between three and five microns, and is less than half the diameter of a red blood cell, capillary diameter will play a major role in determining the resistance to the passage of poorly deformable red cells. In a 1992 paper (66) I suggested

...that subjects with the symptom of tiredness and high percentages of nondiscocytic red cells in their blood, would have smaller-than-usual capillaries, i.e. those with mean capillary diameters falling in the first quartile of a size distribution. Subjects with this characteristic would always be at risk of red-cell-shape related impairment of capillary blood flow. Because of the difficulties of assessing capillary dimensions, it is emphasised that data from red cell shape analysis should not be used in a predictive fashion.

The significance of red cell morphology in the pathogenesis of ME/CFIDS was critiqued by Spurgin (67) who made the interesting observation that the high incidence of ME in women might be a consequence of their having smaller capillaries. She wrote *"Capillary diameter may also explain why women are afflicted not only more frequently but often more severely than men since capillary diameter may be larger in men."* Currently that possibility remains unexplored, but there is little doubt that men have larger muscles than women and for that reason, their blood supply needs could be greater.

Perhaps the most important implication of a concept concerning the possible pathogenicity of shape-changed, poorly deformable red cells is that the use of agents to improve red cell deformability could have therapeutic potential.

However, it needs to be recognised that any activity-related change in red cell shape populations will be additive to any existing change, and it is this feature which may potentiate a relapse. This was well shown by a young woman with ME who brought a blood sample to the office about 9am. On checking the information sheet, I noticed that she considered that she was "well," and pointed out that if she was well it was very likely that the result would be normal. However, late in the afternoon she brought in another blood sample, saying that she had "crashed" about 3.30pm for no apparent reason. After the samples had been assessed, it was found that the first sample was normal and the second sample was very abnormal, which showed very clearly the difference between remission and relapse.

An interesting side issue to the ME story is that in late 1993 I was approached by a high school girl who asked if I could suggest a topic to prepare for a school science fair. I suggested that she should explore the effects of trigger pulling on her own blood, and in addition determine the effects of physiological saline on her blood cells. As this would involve learning how to use the scanning electron microscope, she was very enthusiastic. When she had become proficient in the associated techniques, a blood sample was obtained from a left arm vein. Three drops were fixed immediately and the remainder was added to 5ml of physiological saline. After five minutes in the saline, the red cells were transferred to fixative. She then pulled the trigger of a model revolver until trigger finger fatigue ensued after thirty-five seconds, and the blood sampling procedure was repeated. After overnight fixation, the red cells were processed by a standard technique, gold coated and photographed in the scanning electron microscope. **Red cell shape analysis of the resulting micrographs showed that in her first blood sample there were 10.6% cells**

with altered margins, which increased to 30.4% after 35 seconds of trigger pulling. But after 5 minutes in physiological saline the 10.6% had fallen to 0.9% and the 30.4% had fallen to 0. 4% and the majority of cells were biconcave discocytes. So a school girl's study showed clearly the importance of immediate fixation of red cells in any study of red cell morphology, (68) and possibly of greater importance was the change associated with physiological saline.

An editorial in the British Medical Journal concerning chronic fatigue syndrome and myalgic encephalomyelitis stimulated a good deal of correspondence, which showed the gulf between CFS and ME and those who believe in an organic cause for ME and the opinions of those working in the fields of psychiatry and psychology. Lawrie and Pelosi (69) responded rather aggressively to the critical correspondents and stated that,

> ...patients suffer substantial emotional morbidity, whether the chronic fatigue syndrome is defined by British, or as patients' groups prefer, Australian or American criteria. All three sets of criteria can be used to identify cases on a continuum of fatigue, which includes myalgic encephalomyelitis.

Several statements make it unclear about how they envision the relationship between CFS and ME. For example, they wrote,

> ...but the association between the chronic fatigue syndrome or myalgic encephalomyelitis and psychiatric or psychological problems is indisputable, even though the conditions are not entirely explicable in these terms.

The quoted reference for this information was written by a psychiatrist, and titled "Postviral fatigue syndromes and psychiatry," which does not seem to clarify the situation. The authors wrote,

> The repeated criticism of our editorial and the scientific medical journals – that they are biased toward psychiatric and away from 'organic' aetiological theories – is based on isolated reports of brain imaging and neuroendocrine findings, which have not been replicated and have not controlled for depression and inactivity.

But in 1994 the claim that brain imaging reports have not been replicated, indicated a lack of knowledge of the literature. By ignoring our publications of 1986, 1989 and 1992 concerning changes in blood rheology which could impair cerebral blood flow in ME, the authors appear to believe that brain function is not affected by impaired cerebral blood flow. Yet there are several studies which report reduced regional cerebral blood flow in depressive illnesses.

It is possible that the unreplicated study referred to the paper by Dr. Costa presented at the annual general meeting of the British Nuclear Medicine Society on March 30, 1994. Dr. Costa used SPECT to show that in ME people there was a diffuse reduction in brain blood flow and in the brainstem blood flow was reduced in comparison with patients with depression and healthy subjects. In addition, in the front of the 1992 book on ME/CFS by Hyde, Goldstein and Levine, there are several plates showing SPECT scans in ME/CFS patients. The lack of reference to such information seems to imply that the authors were

106

either unaware of such published information, or that they had chosen to make selective use of the literature. Neither situation reflects the expectations of competence from the authors of a British Medical Journal editorial.

Early in 1995, Simpson (70) wrote,

> *As ME organisations are still prominent in New Zealand, Australia, South Africa, the United Kingdom, the Netherlands and Canada, and recently in Italy, it seems that the American concept of CFS is an example of the world dog being wagged by the American tail. Confusion about the nature of CFS has been compounded by the formation of the American Association for Chronic Fatigue Syndrome. This means that when the term CFS is used it needs to be qualified.*

In 1988 the introduction of "*...a working case definition*" for chronic fatigue syndrome was received with early enthusiasm, although it was soon the topic for critical comment, possibly because the criteria were too inclusive. In attempts to improve the position, case definitions were developed in both Australia and England.

With the objective of testing their suitability, Bates et al (71) classified 805 patients according to the three different criteria. They reported that 61% met the CDC criteria; 56% met the Australian criteria; and 55% met the English criteria. But problems arose when it was found that the laboratory abnormalities in those cases which met the different criteria were similar to those who met none of the case definitions. It was concluded "*These data suggest that more inclusive case definitions may be superior.*"

Late in 1994, Fukuda et al (72) proposed a more inclusive and comprehensive case definition of chronic fatigue syndrome. In recognising the inclusive nature of their case definition, the authors proposed, "*...a strategy for sub-grouping fatigued persons in formal investigations.*" When faced with the objective of comparing like with like, the need to sub-classify CFS patients has also been suggested by others. Maybe ME will eventually appear as one of the sub-classifications. **But what appears strange is that neither the case definitions nor the sub-classes within the case definitions are based upon similarities of aetiology or pathogenesis.**

Publication of the different case definitions stimulated many publications which compared and evaluated the different case definitions as well as inducing readers to express their views in correspondence columns. For example, in the July 1, 1995 issue of the Annals of Internal Medicine, four letters on the topic were published. One writer stated that although the new case criteria were better than the 1988 criteria, "*...the clinical and social need for a definitive diagnostic tool remains largely unmet.*" A letter from physicians associated with an insurance company (73) stated

> *The recent article by Fukuda and colleagues improves the clinical framework for viewing what seems to be an etiologically diverse group of disorders that vary in their course (severity, duration and completeness of recovery). When the authors, citing two studies, inform readers that, "...some persons afflicted by the chronic fatigue syndrome improve with time," but, "...most remain functionally impaired for several years.*

LESLIE O. SIMPSON & NANCY BLAKE

Readers may equate "functionally impaired for....years," with "chronically disabled." Later they wrote

> We believe that the physician who, on making a diagnosis of the syndrome, automatically tells his or her patient to cease working is doing a disservice to the patient......Those who are encouraged to do little more than rest are cut off from actions that our society has traditionally viewed as providing satisfaction and meaning in one's life.

Those comments emphasise the conceptual gap between CFS and ME, as in ME, rest is considered as the cornerstone of treatment, and there is little doubt that a proportion of ME sufferers are functionally impaired to the extent that they are chronically disabled.

> Professor Hooper et al. [9] take a somewhat less charitable view of these statements. Insurance companies have a strong financial interest in having potentially expensive illnesses labelled psychiatric, thus excusing themselves from providing payment for physical disability. The U.K. system for awarding disability benefits has similar strong financial motives for giving ME/CFS a psychiatric label.

A brief article in the British Medical Journal (74) by staff from the Department of Psychology of the University of Edinburgh discussed general practitioners' attitudes to patients with self-diagnosed myalgic encephalomyelitis and reported the results from a simple questionnaire sent to two hundred general practitioners. The analysis of the returned questionnaires showed several interesting attitudes in the respondents. **Treatment appeared to be related to social class of the patient.**

When faced with a wide range of symptoms, whether or not myalgic encephalomyelitis was mentioned, the common response was the prescription of anti-depressants. General practitioners considered that those patients with a self-diagnosis of ME could pose problems of management; take up a lot of time; and be less likely to comply with a suggested treatment plan. The authors concluded that it was not a good idea for patients to tell their general practitioners that they believed they had ME.

The article stimulated several letters to the editor which included reference to the case of a sixty-six year old man with a self-diagnosis of ME, (75) but he was shown to have a hypopituitarism. The authors considered that "*Hypopituitarism should be considered in all patients presenting with non-specific symptoms.*" Martin Arber, chairman of Action for ME contributed a feisty response (76) which concluded

> Finally, the vignettes used in the article do not describe typical cases of myalgic encephalomyelitis. Indeed, one of the psychologists who advise us thought the list of symptoms was more indicative of clinical depression. It is not surprising, therefore, that the doctors responded to the different descriptions in slightly different ways.

Writing as the honorary medical adviser of the ME Association, Dr. Charles Shepherd took the rather unusual step of proposing that findings relating to CFS in the USA were directly relevant to ME (77).

Like Martin Arber, he refuted the proposal that ME organisations encouraged self-diagnosis, and he concluded

> ...if patients are still faced with a general practitioner who 'doesn't believe in myalgic encephalomyelitis,' what option do they have but to make a provisional diagnosis using their own initiative?

A 1996 study concerning the health needs of those with myalgic encephalomyelitis raises so many issues that it deserves special scrutiny (78) At the outset it needs to be stated that it seems that the author has made little attempt to become acquainted with the published literature dealing with myalgic encephalomyelitis. Ramsay's work is not referred to nor is there mention of my work concerning blood rheology in those with ME. Even though the Lancet article by Mukherjee stimulated much discussion, both that article and our 1993 report concerning the effects of exercise on red cell shape were not mentioned. Furthermore, of the twenty-four quoted references, six concerned epidemic outbreaks, and eight papers were written by psychologists or psychiatrists.

In essence, the health needs of ME people were being assessed without reference to the published information which sets out the nature of the disorder. To some extent this was foreshadowed by the first sentence which read *"Myalgic encephalomyelitis (ME) is a mysterious and controversial condition."*

The study was the result of Action for ME requesting the Department of Health to provide, *"...better services and for research into ME as a Health Needs Assessment."* A local man with ME wrote about this, just about the time Wakefield's Department of Public Health was considering its 1993-94 Health Needs Assessment programme. Although the first reactions seemed to be dismissive, it was recognised that

> If people in Wakefield who say they have ME could be objectively shown to have certain health needs, then however they are re-labelled or re-categorised, those health needs should remain.

In a section labelled "Natural history of ME," after an assessment of the historical epidemic outbreaks it was concluded

> It is unlikely that these case-clusters reflect the same entity, as they varied markedly in incubation period, attack rates, clinical picture, demography and speed and completeness of recovery. They also differ from the present day pattern of ME, which is sporadic and epidemic.

Evidently the writer was not impressed by the fact that sporadic cases preceded some of the epidemic outbreaks. If the writer had been aware of Ramsay's work, it is unlikely that the following would have been written:

> The core of ME is the subjective sense of fatigue and fatigability, which cannot be substantiated or refuted by subjective tests, be those neurological, psychological, biochemical or immunological.

Given that the physiological concept of muscle fatigue involves impaired blood flow with inadequate rates of delivery of oxygen, of which the writer seemed unaware, it is not surprising that he failed to mention the SPECT studies which showed reduced regional cerebral blood flow in ME people.

The background knowledge of the writer was not enhanced by his use of ME-CFS, as this could be interpreted as showing that his concept of ME was already confused. Subsequently, after reference to the CDC's case definition of CFS, the term ME-CFS was used only on one occasion. However, it was stated, "...*there is something fundamentally flawed within the concept of ME.*" It would have been more accurate to have considered that the writer's concept of ME was fatally flawed.

Reference was made to a National Task Force, in a "Report from the national task force on chronic fatigue syndrome, (CFS) postviral fatigue syndrome, (PVFS) and myalgic encephalomyelitis (ME)." The title does not indicate that it was a response to Action for ME "...to look just at ME," and there was no indication that the Task Force satisfactorily separated the features of the three syndromes. However, it was noted: "...the syndromes are real, sometimes causing major disability, yet were much misunderstood." In addition, it was stated "Many individuals report that their greatest distress results from the dismissive attitude or outright disbelief shown by their doctors."

But the Task Force did not accept that ME was a distinctive entity; the key to recovery being a balance between rest and recovery, with the rejection of the pathological vs. psychological dichotomy. One is left to wonder about the extent to which the relevant literature had been explored by the Task Force which allowed it to reach such a decision, but it does not augur well for ME people.

After a short section which dealt with the viewpoints of local patients, the views of several physicians were reported. Overall, the opinions on ME by contributing general practitioners were dismissive. A hospital neurologist was quoted as stating, "...*we do not make the diagnosis on any of our patients – at least I don't. In the circumstances I am rather mesmerised to find that you are actually thinking of spending time, money and energy on a non-entity.*"

A section titled, "Health needs arising from ME," included the statement

> Four sets of needs emerged from the present assessments: a medical diagnosis, rest, specific treatment and social care needs. All four are problematic, with conflicting views on their value.

It was stated "People with ME want and need a medical label – '...so that's what's wrong with me.' It implies that the unknown has, at least in part, become known." Later it was noted "To the extent that ME is recognised as a medical condition in the United Kingdom, the demand may be justified. But many clinicians contest it."

However, it should be noted that most of the publicised opposition comes from psychologists and psychiatrists. For example, an Australian group of behavioural scientists considered that the worst prognosis for those with ME involved those cases who believed that there was a physical basis for their disorder.

In discussing the need for rest, which showed the confused beliefs of the writer, the need for rest by ME people was contrasted with the physical activity recommended for those who had suffered a stroke or a myocardial infarction. There is a significant literature which shows that both stroke and heart disease are accompanied by an increase in blood viscosity. Others have shown that light physical activity is accompanied by a reduction in blood viscosity which is of particular relevance to those with strokes and heart attacks. Any discussion about rest in ME usually draws attention to the need for some physical activity and that long term absolute rest is not recommended. Although the comparison of the ME state and post-stroke patients was poorly conceived, it was stated *"Anecdotes abound of individuals with ME relapsing through exertion, but one wonders how many others have languished through excessive inactivity."* As the paper was written three years after we published our report of the effects of trigger finger fatigue in ME people, it would appear that the author seemed determined to emphasise his lack of knowledge of the ME literature and his limited contacts with ME people.

Writing under the heading, "Specific treatments," the author noted that the claimed benefits of Efamol Marine have not been replicated. Perhaps he would not have been so dismissive it he had taken the time to investigate the relevant literature. Evening primrose oil (Efamol) contains about 9% of gammalinolenic acid, which has the capacity to circumvent the problems of a dysfunctional enzyme (delta-6-desaturase) which catalyses cis-linolenic acid to gammalinolenic acid. When taken in sufficient quantities, gammalinolenic acid has been shown to increase significantly the blood levels of prostaglandin E1. In 1974 it was reported that prostaglandin E1 improved the flexibility of red blood cells. So the benefits of evening primrose oil, in doses of at least 4000mg daily, are manifested as improved blood flow. If the author had taken the time to acquaint himself with Ramsay's work, he would have become aware that circulatory impairment is a major factor in the ME scenario. What is important is that there are other agents (such as Trental – pentoxifylline) which have similar beneficial effects on blood flow.

In a consideration of "Social care needs", given the writer's lack of understanding of the nature of ME, it was not surprising that he wrote

> *The present study cannot define the social care needs of people with ME, which should be related to the degree of disability or debility rather than to the condition causing it.*

The summary included the statement

> *...all four categories of need of people with ME are highly debatable. Its diagnosis does not lead to better understanding of cause, management and prognosis. The optimum degree of rest is uncertain. No specific medical treatments are proven. Social care needs have not been quantified but will reflect level of disability rather than causative condition The implication is that there are no health needs arising from ME for which the health authority should purchase or commission services.*

In other words, because people have an illness which is not understood by the medical profession, there is no requirement to consider their social care needs. What an extraordinary situation!

Amongst other things in the conclusions it was stated "What this means in Wakefield is that people with ME continue to receive whatever general primary or secondary care their doctor thinks appropriate." Later it was noted

> *The purchaser will, however, be sceptical of anything that reinforces the idea of ME as a separate mysterious illness. We will probably decline to fund extra-contractual referrals, e.g. for SPECT scans or to fringe practitioners.*

As the SPECT scan study by Costa, referred to previously, had revealed a generalised reduction in brain perfusion, it is strange that a test which had shown a specific pathophysiological change would not be funded.

'It is strange that a test which had shown a specific pathophysiological change would not be funded'. This is strange only if you credit the author with a genuine concern for gaining an understanding of this illness. It isn't strange at all for a person whose agenda is to dismiss ME as psychological in order to decline funding for a test which would prove that ME has clear-cut, measurable physical effects. Refusing to do tests which would show physical effects, such as the Tilt test, which would indicate reduced blood flow, continues to be the advice provided by NICE for the guidance of physicians dealing with patients suffering from ME, because wanting such tests is simply another indication of our insistence on having a physical diagnosis. This perfectly reasonable insistence is labelled as yet another symptom of the fact that ME is 'somatoform'.

The author concluded

> *If purchasers are to become sceptical about ME, and urge clinicians to restrict themselves to evidence-based intervention, then equal scepticism should apply to the purchasing function. The concept of ME is under assault, but it may outlast the concept of purchasing.*

While the extent to which this official's attitude will disadvantage ME people can only be guessed at, it seems that it is justifiable to adopt a, "don't confuse me with facts – my mind's made up" attitude. If the Wakefield situation is reflected in other English communities, then those who have the health-related problems of suffering from ME will be disadvantaged by the lack of social and health-related services.

An important event concerning the publicising of our activities occurred on December 5, 1996 when I spoke to an ME audience at an evening meeting in Victoria, British Columbia. After question time, I was approached by Dr. Abram Hoffer, who introduced himself as the editor of the Journal of Orthomolecular Medicine. He invited me to contribute a written version of the lecture he had just heard. So, in the middle of 1997, a paper titled, "Myalgic encephalomyelitis (ME): a haemorheological disorder manifested as impaired capillary blood flow" (79) was published. The paper concluded

> *My interest in ME is based solely upon a desire to help a section of the community who suffer from a debilitating illness which has yet to gain acceptance from the medical community. At the risk of being considered irrational about the biological importance of normal capillary blood flow, I can point with satisfaction to the*

many ME patients who have benefited from treatment with haemorheological agents.

Later in the year, the same journal published a report of the red cell shape analysis results from nearly 2200 blood samples from members of ME groups in four countries (80).

> The following paragraphs discuss the problems of classification and the implications of the variety of terms used, some of which may include ME along with other illnesses, and others may exclude ME altogether, while purporting to have relevance to it.

In December 2001, Marshall, Williams and Hooper (81) published a booklet containing information for clinicians and lawyers, titled, "What is ME? What is CFS?" An insert stated *"This booklet contains condensed information which was supplied to the Working Group on CFS-ME, but was ignored by them."* A peculiar feature of the publication is that the results of studies involving Americans with CFS are equated with ME. Apparently, this is on the basis that, *"Chronic Fatigue Syndrome (CFS) is listed in ICD-10 as a term by which ME is also known, as is the term Postviral Fatigue Syndrome (PVFS). The term "CFIDS" or Chronic Fatigue and Immune Dysfunction Syndrome, is used by some groups in the US."* It would seem that the continued use of ME/ICD-CFS rather than ME is based upon the premise of legitimacy through the WHO classification. However, as ME is classified as a neurological disorder, and neurological problems are only one part of the disorder, it is uncertain if anything has been gained with the name change.

Although some of Ramsay's papers and letters are quoted, no mention is made of the second edition of his book, in which he placed ME symptoms into three groups: muscle phenomena, circulatory impairment and cerebral dysfunction. While ME/ICD-CFS provided protection against claims that the problem was psychological or psychiatric, it seems to have inhibited discussion about the Ramsay criteria and their implications. As an example, not one of the one hundred and seventy-two quoted references specifically investigated the "circulatory impairment," quoted by Ramsay, apart from some neuro-imaging studies which showed reduced regional cerebral blood flow. **But such reports never discuss possible causes for the reduced cerebral blood flow**. Yet, although none of our reports concerning changes in the blood flow properties of ME were referred to, those studies would have provided a basis for understanding the changes in cerebral blood flow.

This obvious rejection of the Ramsay criteria led to some rather unexpected conclusions. For example, although the aetiology of ME remains unexplained, it was stated, *"Specifically, the mechanism of the incapacitating exhaustion is identical in the two conditions (i.e. in ME and in Post-Polio Syndrome)."* The discussion on "Symptoms," stated, *"In ME, symptoms are seemingly without end. There is a remarkable variability of signs and symptoms from day to day and even from hour to hour."* Even though there are very few statements about remissions in CFS, it was noted, *"The waxing and waning in the same patients in the same day is typical of almost all findings in ME/ICD-CFS, and may lead to medical scepticism."* A very extensive list of symptoms was quoted with one reference to CFIDS patients. It was stated *"There may be significant and permanent damage to skeletal and cardiac muscles as well as other end organs, etc."* But there is no published evidence of such pathology, post-mortem, in ME people, and it is not possible to imagine permanent tissue damage associated with symptoms which waxed and waned. Furthermore, if such symptoms were identifiable, then histological analysis could reveal something of their pathogenesis.

In a discussion of "Evidence of abnormalities in ME," it was stated that there was evidence of inflammation of the central nervous system, but *"Such inflammation is not found in all variants of CFS."* It was not made clear what relationship existed between "abnormalities of ME", and "variants of CFS". While it was claimed that there was *"... some degree of encephalitis in ME"* it was not explained how remissions could occur during encephalitis and inflammation of the central nervous system. Maybe it was not surprising that the reference to that conclusion was the opinion of an American expert on CFS, even though the section was headed "Evidence of abnormalities in ME." The American expert, (Dr. A. L. Komaroff) in an article published in 2000 with the title, "The biology of chronic fatigue syndrome," had concluded

> *In summary, there is now considerable evidence of an underlying biological process in most patients (which) is inconsistent with the hypothesis that (the syndrome) involves symptoms that are only major or amplified because of underlying psychiatric distress. It is time to put that hypothesis to rest.*

In 1988 Dr. Komaroff was one of the group who formalised the CFS guidelines, making CFS a much more inclusive diagnosis than ME. If there is evidence of abnormalities in ME people, this was not clearly established.

A section titled, "Precipitating factors" contained some new concepts, in which three precipitating events were identified: stress, toxic exposure and physical trauma *"particularly a motor vehicle accident."* But in the two hundred and seventy-four ME groups that I have spoken to in six countries, I have never met an ME person who claimed that a vehicle accident was the cause of their ME. In addition it was claimed that bacterial and viral infections, vaccinations and anaesthetics caused the disorder to worsen.

Rather surprisingly, there was no reference to the three factors which precipitated relapses commonly referred to in the reports of epidemic outbreaks, namely, physical activity, cold weather and the onset of menstruation. Some reports also mentioned vaccinations. The significance of the precipitating factors is that they all have an adverse influence on blood rheology. There are several reports of the fatal effects of cold weather which increases blood viscosity, but all of the other factors stimulate changes in the shape populations of red blood cells, which is associated with reduced red cell deformability and impairment of blood flow in the microcirculation. Individuals with an existing change in their red cell shape populations (such as in ME) are most adversely affected, because the effects of a precipitating factor are additive to the existing change, resulting in an exacerbation of their symptoms.

When considering "Physical signs found in ME," the authors quoted a long list of symptoms, but there was no mention of Ramsay's three cardinal signs, which could be another indication that Ramsay's contribution to the understanding of ME was being disregarded.

It is strange that under this heading, Dr. Paul Cheney was recognised as "*...one of the world's leading exponents of ME/ICD-CFS,*" who quoted his experience with CFS in detail. Although many high technology test results were quoted, in no test was there 100% positivity. What is uncertain is how Dr. Cheney's results relate to ME, but it is unlikely that the authors would have recognised the irony in their statement, "*Despite all this authenticated international research, much of the current perception of ME, both medical and lay, is beset by confusion and misinformation.*"

No mention of our published papers was made in the one hundred and seventy-two quoted references, even though we had addressed the effects of exercise on red cell shape and blood flow. Because SPECT scans will be influenced by factors which influence blood flow, the possible relationship between poorly filterable blood and SPECT-demonstrated reduced regional cerebral blood flow was not considered. But until the effects of impaired microcirculatory blood flow are incorporated into the natural history of ME, "confusion and misinformation" will persist.

Given the authors' apparent acceptance of ME as a synonym for CFS, the section, "Changing definitions: history of chronic fatigue syndrome (CFS)," has some interesting statements. The section began "*In the US in the late 1970s and 1980s there seemed to be a remarkable rise in incidence of a condition indistinguishable from ME, with manifestations of serious neuro-immune disease and profound incapacity, etc.*" **Because there is no National Health Service in the US, the health insurance industry became concerned, noting that "*...the field could change from an epidemiological investigation into a health insurance nightmare.*" It was alleged that the insurance industry influenced the development of a new case definition which was so worded that insurers would not be liable.** The authors stated

'CFS' did not come into existence until 1988. As a basis for sound scientific research it has been a disaster. 'CFS' is not a single diagnostic entity and 'fatigue' is not a disorder, it is a symptom. The term 'CFS,' is now applied to a heterogeneous group, as a non-specific label, which embraces many different medical and psychiatric conditions, in which tiredness and fatigue are prominent.

This is an excellent summary of the significance of CFS. It is of interest that two members of the expert panel which produced the 1988 guidelines, refused to sign the final version, "*...because the proposed definition and new name were so different from the ME with which they were so familiar.*"

Five-and-a-half of the twenty pages of text were devoted to a discussion of "How 'CFS' displaced ME in the UK" which details the various actions of the Wessely School in a campaign to abolish ME, and included the idea that ME related to those, "*...who seek treatment rather than those who suffer the symptoms.*" It was stated "*Wessely's determination to eradicate ME as a legitimate medical entity never seems to cease.*" In general the status of the Wessely School was not enhanced by an attempt to change the WHO classification of ME from neurological to psychiatric, but it provides a good indication of the strength of the views held by the School. The most obvious feature of the controversial situation is the confusion concerning the relevant nomenclature. The authors stated in bold *"It is important to be familiar with the fact that 'chronic fatigue' and chronic 'fatigue syndromes' do not equate with chronic fatigue syndrome (CFS) or with ME."*

Buried under the mess of the name controversy is the fact that it is a change in the internal environment, caused by a variety of factors, which on the one hand may lead to remission, or on the other hand lead to an exacerbation of symptoms. Reference was made to suggested name changes such as Neuro-endocrine Immune Dysfunction Syndrome and Chronic Neuroendocrine Dysfunction Syndrome, but both titles stimulate the question, *"What is the cause (or causes) of the dysfunctional state?"*

As far as ME sufferers in the UK are concerned, the continuing activities of the Wessely School do not augur well for their future wellbeing. As an advisor to the government Dr. Wessely has a great deal of influence which is manifested in his ability to attract funding from a wide range of sources for his research. His influence at the highest political and commercial levels will be sure to have an adverse effect on the extent to which the health needs of ME people are delivered.

It would be highly desirable for every politician, physician and ME sufferer in the UK, to be provided with a copy of "How 'CFS' displaced ME in the UK" so that the public at large could learn how in this debate, matters relating to scientific method are diluted and not clearly separated from political influence. As psychiatry is not a science, and therefore is unable to measure symptoms or to define their cause, it seems strange that a group of psychiatrists should wield such enormous influence in the field of ME. It can only be hoped that in the end science will prevail and the irrelevance of psychiatry to ME will be established conclusively.

My last contribution to the ME literature was a short paper titled, "On the pathophysiology of ME/CFS," published in 2000. (82) The title reflected editorial opinion. As many ME people complain that "…they feel old" it is relevant that a study of blood samples from healthy subjects aged between 60 and 96 years, showed that the aging process was accompanied by high values for flat cells, which is the same change which occurs in chronic ME (83). For that reason it is not surprising that age-related problems such as cold hands and feet, muscle weakness and memory problems occur also in ME people.

In 2007 the Journal of Clinical Pathology published a series of papers, two of which used myalgic encephalomyelitis in the title. Puri (82) discussed the role of long-chain polyunsaturated fatty acids in the pathophysiology of myalgic encephalomyelitis, with chronic fatigue syndrome as a synonym. It is strange that no reference was made to the work of David Horrobin who had published in the same field many years earlier, so it is not surprising that their findings were not different. The author wrote

> *These findings (of immune system changes) are consistent with those of a pre-existing, long-term viral infection. Although these findings are also consistent with an autoimmune response, there is little evidence to support this possibility in myalgic encephalomyelitis.*

Such a statement implies that the writer was unaware that no study of ME people has shown a 100% incidence of a viral infection, or that there is a small proportion of ME people with a non-infective prelude to their development of ME. It would also need to be explained how remissions could occur during long-term infection.

As his findings are not new, it could be significant that he referred to a commercial product which is based on, "...*virgin, cold-pressed, non-raffinated evening primrose oil,*" and "...*ultra-pure eicosapentaenoic acid,*" (VegEPA) with a daily dose of between two and eight capsules daily. Because of the costs of refinement, it is unlikely that the new product will be cheap, so it is relevant that Horrobin showed that four grams daily of evening primrose oil produced a significant increase in the blood levels of prostaglandin E1. In 1974 it had been shown the prostaglandin E1 improved red cell flexibility. Furthermore, it would not have been unreasonable to have learned how the action of VegEPA compared with the published effects of fish oil, which contains eicosapentaenoic acid. One of those studies showed that sardine oil improved red cell membrane flexibility and thus increased the rate of capillary blood flow.

Moreover, Puri gave no indication that he was aware of the published information concerning the flow problems of ME blood, or of Ramsay's concept of "circulatory impairment." But there is no quarrel with the conclusion *"Treatment with long-chain polyunsaturated acids may offer a potential therapeutic route,"* as this has been shown previously.

While it would be encouraging to think that by 2007 there would be a better understanding of ME, unfortunately that is not the case and to demonstrate how concepts can be rendered unintelligible, reference is made to a paper from Canada (85), the title of which commences, "Definitions and aetiology of myalgic encephalomyelitis." The paper contains sixteen quoted references, most of which have little relevance to ME. It is far from clear just what message was being delivered, as the paper is marked by the use of complexly-worded concepts, frequently embedded in sentences of more than fifty words. Towards the end of the paper, reference to the aetiology was noted as *"The possible aetiology of myalgic encephalomyelitis is under scientific observation"* just as it has been since the 1970s. In conclusion it was stated

> *The problem of cultivating a holistic view without adequately structuring the field with a proper clinical entity can lead to great confusions of relevance, where contextual and syndromal features are confounded, with no way of clinically quantifying their relative effects. Choose the right kind of entity or you may end up only considering background factors with no clinical entity left that they are the background of – see the fate of the Cheshire cat in 'Alice in Wonderland.' where the cat fades leaving only the smile.*

While it is possible that the quotation of 'Alice in Wonderland,' might have wider connotations, it is far from clear just what message the conclusion was meant to convey, and individual readers are invited to try and relate the statement to their personal concept of ME.

On January 29, 2007, The Nightingale Research Foundation published a report written by Dr. B. Hyde in response to a request by Dr. Ian Gibson, as chairman of the joint committee on ME in the House of Commons. The report was titled, "The Nightingale Myalgic Encephalomyelitis (M.E.) Definition."

In the "Preface" it was stated, "…there has been a tendency by some individuals and organizations to assume that M.E. and CFS are the same illness," and that there should be name changes. But it was noted "This does not seem to me to be a useful initiative; it would simply add credence to the mistaken assumption that M.E. and CFS represent the same disease process. They do not. M.E. is a clearly defined disease process. CFS by definition has always been a syndrome."

After criticising the widespread use of CFS as a "psychiatric label," and the CDC guidelines, the author wrote, "To my knowledge, **in the entire history of medicine, there are simply no disease definitions that have been assembled with a structure similar to the CFS definition.**"

Prior to the presentation of the Nightingale Definition of M.E., it was stated "I believe it essential to define clearly, Myalgic Encephalomyelitis, returning the definition to its clinical and historic roots and complementing this information WITH THE CERTITUDE OF MODERN SCIENTIFIC TESTING" (my emphasis). As the second edition of Ramsay's book is in the cited references, it might have been expected that Ramsay's views would have equated with "…clinical and historic roots" but this is not the case.

The Definition of M.E. is given as

> *Primary M.E. is an acute onset, epidemic or endemic (sporadic) infectious disease process, where there is always a measurable and persistent diffuse vascular injury of the CNS in both the acute and chronic phases. Primary M.E. is associated with immune and other pathologies.*

Note the implications of the phrase, "…*measurable and persistent diffuse vascular injury of the CNS, etc.*," as this appears to have been based upon neuroimaging studies. However, without mention of remissions or relapses, can it be claimed that the definition has returned to its historic roots? For example, compare the definition with that of Ramsay, who in the second edition of his book (87) stated

> *The clinical entity of myalgic encephalomyelitis syndrome rests on three distinct features namely:*
>
> 1. *a unique form of muscle fatigability whereby, even after a minor degree of physical effort, three four or five days, or longer, may elapse before full muscle power is restored;*
> 2. *variability and fluctuations of both symptoms and physical findings in the course of a day; and*
> 3. *an alarming tendency to become chronic.*

And in his discussion on the endemic nature of ME, Ramsay subdivided the problem into muscle phenomena, circulatory impairment and cerebral dysfunction. The two definitions are so different that it is difficult to imagine the same disorder is involved. Note also that Ramsay (and others) referred to the "ME Syndrome," whereas Hyde considered that "M.E.

is a clearly defined disease process." But if it is a clearly defined process, why has the topic stimulated such antagonism from psychiatrists and why is it so controversial?

At least superficially, Hyde's concept of, "...*certitude of modern scientific testing*," is based upon his neuroimaging studies, in which he interprets reduced regional cerebral blood flow in terms of vascular damage. However, there are other chronic disorders which show reduced regional cerebral blood flow under SPECT scans. For example, this occurs in depressive illnesses. One study reported that in a region where blood flow was reduced during depression, it was normal after the resolution of the depression. **Such an observation indicates that a concept of vascular damage is untenable and would reinforce the possibility that the observed changes were explicable in terms of capillary dimension and reduced red cell deformability.** If small capillaries were randomly distributed, then they would become important determinants of blood flow in the presence of poorly deformable red cells. The evidence which supports this proposal is embodied in SPECT studies which record that post exercise scans show reduced rates of blood flow in comparison with the pre-exercise state. Energetic activity changes the shape populations of red cells, with an associated reduction in the deformability of such cells, and will reduce the rate of capillary blood flow.

As has been stated elsewhere, the great variability of symptoms among ME people could be indicators of the presence of clusters of small capillaries. Such a proposal is supported by the results from a SPECT study of patients suffering from one of three different psychiatric disorders. The results showed that different regions of the brain had reduced rates of blood flow in each of the three disorders. Such a finding is consistent with the idea that normal rates of blood flow and oxygen delivery are needed to sustain normal brain function.

As muscle fatigability and symptom variability during a short time span were not discussed by Hyde, the nature of the clinical and historic roots to which he alluded remains uncertain.

A primary problem concerning reports of SPECT scans is that they lack discussions concerning the cause of the problem and how they might be treated. **Although Hyde considers that vascular damage and vasculitis are involved, such a concept implies irreversible change, but given time, the post-exercise reduction in regional cerebral blood flow returns to normal. Therefore, it could be anticipated that when treated with agents which increase red cell deformability, SPECT scans should show improved regional cerebral blood flow.** An investigation of the relevant literature showed that there are many published studies which show improved regional cerebral blood flow in both animals and man after treatment with agents which improve blood flow and red cell deformability, such as pentoxifylline. However no report commented on the effects of the drug on red cell deformability, but Dormehl et al (88) reported that in healthy volunteers aged between fifty-two and seventy years, after two months of treatment with pentoxifylline (800mg) and nicotinic acid (200mg) daily, there was a pronounced improvement in cerebral blood flow, particularly in the frontal and cerebellar regions. Participants spontaneously volunteered the information that their memory and general well-being had improved.

The Differing Concepts of ME.

In a brief paper titled, "What is ME?" ME Research UK stated, "Myalgic encephalomyelitis (ME) is characterised by a range of neurological symptoms and signs, muscle pain with intense physical or mental exhaustion, relapses and specific cognitive disabilities." However, there was no recognition of the remissions which Ramsay had reported in the second edition of his book. In any multi-system disorder, it is worth noting that the various tissues are linked by both the nervous system and the blood vascular system. This carries the implication that the primary cause of multi-system dysfunction could reside in either system. But normal functioning of the nervous system is dependent upon the availability of normal levels of oxygen, yet this may not occur if capillary blood flow is impaired.

It was noted that during relapses, "…fresh episodes of muscle weakness" or "…well defined cognitive problems," may develop.

According to physiology textbooks, muscle weakness or muscle fatigue is a consequence of an inadequate supply of oxygen as a result of a reduced rate of blood flow. Furthermore, cognitive dysfunction has been shown by SPECT scans to be associated with reduced regional cerebral blood flow.

It was unfortunate that the term "fatigue" was introduced, without definition, together with the claim that fatigue in ME patients is different from the fatigue experienced by healthy subjects. This situation was not made any clearer when in a list of "Key facts," it was stated, *"Characteristic symptoms include muscle pain with physical and mental exhaustion following normal activities; quite different from what is normally experienced by healthy people."* This seems to equate "fatigue" with "exhaustion", when tiredness might have been a better term.

As our published work concerning impaired blood flow in ME was not referred to, it is not surprising that the paper concluded, *"The cause is still unknown, and no cure or effective treatment has yet been found."*

In marked contrast to the views expressed by the UK group, American ME groups seem to consider that changing the name to ME from CFS is simply a word game. In January 2007, a CFS Name-Change Advisory Board, which consisted of investigators who had been involved with CFS research for some years, decided that in the future, CFS would be known as ME.

A relevant web page began

> *The ME Society of America is an organisation that seeks to promote understanding of the disease known as myalgic encephalomyelitis (ME/CFS), a multisystem disease that adversely affects the cellular mitochondria, and the heart, brain, neuroendocrine, immune and circulatory systems.*

Later it was stated, "Dr. A Melvin Ramsay outlined a definitional framework for ME that described abnormal muscle metabolism, circulatory impairment and cerebral involvement." The conjunction of these two statements was probably meant to show that Ramsay's work had been considered, but there was no mention of the remissions which Ramsay had described and which were central to his concept of ME. In a rather puzzling statement, it was noted

> *The ME Society of America (MESA) website features research and advocacy issues pertaining to ME and ME/CFS as it is defined by the Canadian Clinical Case Definition and by the Holmes et al case definition for CFS, and does not represent patients with so-called "CFS" as it is currently defined by the U.S. Centers for Disease Control and Prevention.*

The problem is that both the Canadian case definition and the Holmes et al definitions do not recognise Ramsay's concept.

As will be discussed later, the Canadian Guidelines have a very controversial approach to ME, and in the introduction to their paper, the authors stated, *"Myalgic encephalomyelitis and chronic fatigue syndrome are used interchangeably and this disease is referred to as ME/CFS."* This is the probable explanation for the use of ME/CFS throughout the MESA website, and in the "Definitional framework" it is stated, *"M.E. and CFS are not two different diseases (even if there are two different case definitions)."*

A section titled, "M.E. is not "Medically Unexplained", contains the statement

> *Circulatory impairment, which the CDC case definition fails to mention, has been explained in terms of coagulopathy (Berg) and/or abnormal erythrocyte morphology (Simpson) low plasma/erythrocyte volume (Streeten) and low cardiac output (Cheney).*

However, the author has failed to recognise the importance of the different red cell shape populations and that the different red cell shapes are not evidence of abnormal erythrocyte morphology, as they occur in normal blood. **In relation to ME, the importance of the different red cell shape populations is that they return to normal during remissions**.

According to MESA, "The most compelling research to date that explains the severe physical dysfunctionality in ME/CFS is the research on low cardiac output." But it would be impossible to explain ME remissions which may last for hours or days in terms of a low cardiac output.

The section on "Etiology" is interesting, and commences

> *ME/CFS appears to be a different insult/same result disease, and no single viral, bacterial, or environmental etiology is likely to be found, although we are open to any discovery to the contrary. However, as Ramsay states 'The particular invading microbial agent is probably not the most important factor...the key to the problem is likely to be found in the abnormal response of the patient to the organism.*

The section concluded, *"While the insults may be different, there may be a common pathophysiology."* It should be emphasised that the factor in common for infections, or toxins or emotional upsets etc., is that they induce changes in the internal environment which in turn stimulates changes in the shape populations of red blood cells. Because blood containing changed red cell shape populations is poorly filterable, there will be increased resistance to blood flow in the microcirculation.

So it is very relevant that in 1989, Dr. Ann Macintyre wrote

It is probable that during a relapse, there is something wrong with the red blood cells, making it harder for them to travel along the smallest vessels (capillaries) to supply oxygen to the tissues... the red blood cells become abnormally shaped during a relapse, losing their biconcave, smooth disc-like appearance... These findings would explain the poor microcirculation and poor oxygenation of tissues and hence the impaired removal of by-products of metabolism, such as lactic acid, from the tissues.

Therefore, in terms of Ramsay's concept of the importance of the patient's response, and Macintyre's idea of poor microcirculation, the response would be most different in patients with smaller than usual capillaries who would manifest the symptoms of ME.

It is difficult to accept MESA's concept of research into people with CFS being relevant to Ramsay's concept of ME, which was diagnosed by excluding other possible diagnoses. For example, if heart dysfunction was involved, then a diagnosis of ME would be excluded.

According to the NAME website:

The National Alliance for Myalgic Encephalomyelitis (NAME US) was established to address the issues of recognition and definition, and to raise awareness of this devastating neuroimmune disease that has afflicted nearly a million people in the US and millions worldwide.

The Introduction commences

Myalgic encephalomyelitis (M.E.) is a neurological disease with serious CNS consequences due to brain injury, with serious cardiovascular and immunological consequences. M.E. is a clear-cut definitional diagnosis with tests that can show the effects of M.E. such as: SPECT and PET scans, Natural Killer Cell Function Test, RNA-ase anti-viral dysregulation, and Blood Flow

Clearly the NAME concept has little relationship to Ramsay's concept of ME, and it is noteworthy that remissions are not mentioned. Having studied the occurrence of remissions in patients with a physician's diagnosis of ME, it is not possible to accept that such patients had a neuroimmune disorder. Therefore it would seem that the condition diagnosed as ME in the 1980s and earlier, is not the same as the condition being investigated in the USA in the 21st century, even though it has been given the same name.

Chapter III References

1. Anonymous. Lancet 1956: 1:789 (Editorial).
2. Anonymous. Epidemic myalgic encephalomyelitis. Br Med J 1957; 2: 927-8.
3. Medical Staff, Royal Free Hospital. An outbreak of encephalomyelitis in the Royal Free Hospital Group, London, in 1955. Br Med J 1957; 2: 895-904.
4. Price JL. Myalgic encephalomyelitis. Lancet 1961; 1: 737-8.
5. McEvedy CP, Beard AW. Royal Free epidemic of 1955: a reconsideration. Br Med J 1970; 1: 7-11.
6. McEvedy AW, Beard AW. Concept of benign myalgic encephalomyelitis. Br Med J 1970; 1: 11-15.

7. Innes SGB. Encephalomyelitis resembling benign myalgic encephalomyelitis. Lancet 1970; 1: 969-71
8. Lyle WH. Encephalomyelitis resembling benign myalgic encephalomyelitis. Lancet; 1: 1118-9. (Letter)
9. Parish JG. Benign myalgic encephalomyelitis. Brit J Psychiatr 1973: 122: 735. (Letter)
10. Ramsay AM, Dowsett EG, Dadswell JV et al. Icelandic disease (benign myalgic encephalomyelitis or Royal Free Disease). Br Med J 1977; 1: 1350. (Letter)
11. Anonymous. Epidemic myalgic encephalomyelitis. Br Med J 1978; 1: 1436-7 (Editorial).
12. Behan PO. Post-infection encephalomyelitis: some aetiological mechanisms. Postgrad Med J 1978; 54: 755-9.
13. Church AJ. Myalgic encephalomyelitis, "An obscene cosmic joke." Med J Aust 1980; 1: 307-8.
14. Bishop J. Epidemic myalgic encephalomyelitis. Med J Aust 1980; 1: 585-7.
15. Church AJ. Myalgic encephalomyelitis. Med J Aust 1980; 2: 224.(Letter)
16. Miller SE, Roses AD, Appel SH. Scanning electron microscope studies in muscular dystrophy. Arch Neurol 1976; 33:172-4.
17. May PGR, Donnan SPB, Ashton JR, et al. Personality and medical perception in benign myalgic encephalomyelitis. Lancet 1981; 1: 37 (Letter).
18. Goodwin CS. Was it benign myalgic encephalomyelitis? Lancet 1981;1: 37. (Letter)
19. May PGR, Donnan SPB, Ashton JR, et al. Was it benign myalgic encephalomyelitis? Lancet 1981; 1:37-8 (letter).
20. Gow PJ. Myalgic encephalomyelitis. NZ Med J 1984; 97:620 (Letter).
21. Snow P. Myalgic encephalomyelitis. NZ Med J 1984; 97:698 (Letter).
22. Simpson LO, Shand BI, Olds RJ. Myalgic encephalomyelitis. NZ Med J 1984; 87:698-9 (Letter).
23. Gow PJ. Myalgic encephalomyelitis. NZ Med J 1984; 97:868 (Letter).
24. Matthew C. Myalgic encephalomyelitis. NZ Med J 1984; 782 (Letter).
25. Simpson LO, Shand BI, Olds RJ. Myalgic encephalomyelitis. NZ Med J 1986; 98:20 (Letter).
26. Gow PJ. Myalgic encephalomyelitis. NZ Med J 1985; 98:20 (Letter).
27. Murdoch JC. Myalgic encephalomyelitis. NZ Med J 1985; 98:20-1(Letter).
28. Staines D. Myalgic encephalomyelitis hypothesis. Med J Aust 1985; 1143:91 (Letter).
29. Simpson LO, Shand BI, Olds RJ. Blood rheology and myalgic encephalomyelitis: a pilot study. Pathology 1986; 18:190-2.
30. Mukherjee TM, Smith K, Maros K. Abnormal red-blood-cell morphology in myalgic encephalomyelitis. Lancet 1987; 2:328-9 (Letter).
31. Vasilvejic ZM, Polic DD. Morphological changes of erythrocytes in patients and carriers of Duchenne disease. Acta Neurol Scand 1983; 67:242-4.

32. Markesbery WR, Butterfield DA. Scanning electron microscope studies of erythrocytes in Huntington's Disease. Biochem Biophys Res Commun 1977; 78:560-4.

33. Yasuda Y, Akiguchi I, Shio H, et al. Scanning electron microscopy studies of erythrocytes in spinocerebellar degeneration. J Neurol Neurosurg Psychiatry 1984; 47:269-74.

34. Pantely GA, Swenson LJ, Tamblyn CH, et al. Increased vascular resistance to a reduction in red cell deformability in the isolated hind limb of swine. Microvasc Res 1988; 35:86-100.

35. Kon K, Maeda N, Ishiga T. The influence of deformation of transformed erythrocytes during flow on the rate of oxygen release. J Physiol 1983; 339:573-84.

36. Vandergrif KD, Olson JS. Morphological and physical factors affecting oxygen uptake and release by red blood cells. J Biol Chem 1984; 259:12619-27.

37. Murdoch JC. Myalgic encephalomyelitis syndrome – an analysis of the findings in 200 cases. NZ Fam Phys 1987; 14:51-4.

38. Byrne E. Idiopathic chronic fatigue and myalgia syndrome (myalgic encephalomyelitis): some thoughts on nomenclature and aetiology. Med J Aust 1988; 148:80-2.

39. Byrne E. Pathophysiology of myalgic encephalomyelitis. Med J Aust 1988; 148:598 (Letter).

40. Bell EJ, McCartney RA, Riding MH. Coxsackie B virus and myalgic encephalomyelitis. J Roy Soc Med 1988; 81:329-31.

41. Lloyd AR, Wakefield D, Broughton C, et al. What is myalgic encephalomyelitis? Lancet 1988; 1:1286-7 (Letter).

42. Ramsay AM. Myalgic encephalomyelitis or what? Lancet 1988; 2:100 (Letter).

43. Dowsett EG. Myalgic encephalomyelitis or what? Lancet 1988; 2:101 (Letter).

44. David AS, Wessely S, Pelosi AJ. Myalgic encephalomyelitis or what? Lancet 1988; 2:100-1 (Letter).

45. Murdoch JC. The myalgic encephalomyelitis syndrome. Fam Pract 1988; 5:302-6.

46. Simpson LO. Nondiscocytic erythrocytes in myalgic encephalomyelitis. NZ Med J 1989; 102:126-7.

47. Wessely S. Myalgic encephalomyelitis – a warning: discussion paper. J Roy Soc Med 1989; 82:215-7.

48. Richmond C. Myalgic encephalomyelitis, Princess Aurora and the wandering womb. Br Med J 1989; 298:1295-6.

49. Coakley JH. Myalgic encephalomyelitis and muscle fatigue. Br Med J 1989; 298:1295-6.

50. Griffiths M. Introduction to Human Physiology. MacMillan Publishing Company Inc., New York, 1981, pp 73-4.

51. WiLes CM, Jones DA, Edwards RHT. Fatigue in human metabolic myopathy. Ciba Foundation Symposium 1981; 82:264-82.

52. Murdoch JC. The myalgic encephalomyelitis syndrome. NZ Med J 1989; 102:372-3.

53. Snow P. Myalgic encephalomyelitis. NZ Med J 1989; 102:449 (Letter).
54. Spracklen FH. The chronic fatigue syndrome (myalgic encephalomyelitis) myth or mystery? South Afr Med J 1988; 74:448-52.
55. Lev M. Myalgic encephalomyelitis. J Roy Soc Med 1989; 82:693-4 (Letter).
56. Rose E, Jagannath P, Wessely S. Possible ME. The Practitioner 1990; 234:195-8.
57. Prasher D, Smith A, Findley L. Sensory and cognitive event-related potentials in myalgic encephalomyelitis. J Neurol Neurosurg Psychiatry 1990; 53:247-53.
58. Lynch S, Seth R. Depression and myalgic encephalomyelitis. J Roy Soc Med 1990; 83:341(Letter).
59. Dowsett EG, Ramsay AM, McCartney RA, et al. Myalgic encephalomyelitis – a persistent viral infection. Postgrad Med J 1990; 66:526-30.
60. Wilson CWM. Myalgic encephalomyelitis: an alternative hypothesis. J Roy Soc Med 1990; 83:481-3 (Editorial).
61. Wessely S. Myalgic encephalomyelitis. J Roy Soc Med 1991; 84:182 (Letter).
62. Simpson LO. The role of nondiscocytic erythrocytes in the pathogenesis of myalgic encephalomyelitis. In: Hyde BM, Goldstein J, Levine P (eds). The clinical and scientific basis of myalgic encephalomyelitis/chronic fatigue syndrome. The Nightingale Research Foundation, Ottawa, 1992, pp597-605.
63. Hume MC. Self-help organisation's advice on myalgic encephalomyelitis. Br Med J 1992; 305:649 (Letter)
64. Simpson LO, Murdoch JC, Herbison GP. Red cell shape changes following trigger finger fatigue in subjects with chronic tiredness and healthy controls. NZ Med J 1993; 106:104-7.
65. Tanahashi N, Meyer JS, Ishikawa Y, et al. Cerebral blood flow and cognitive testing correlate in Huntington's Disease. Arch Neurol 1985; 42:1169-75.
66. Simpson LO. Chronic tiredness and idiopathic chronic fatigue – a connection? NJMed 1992; 89:211-6
67. Spurgin M. The role of red blood cell morphology in the pathogenesis of M.E./CFIDS. CFIDS Chronicle 1995; Summer: 55-8.
68. Simpson. Red cell shape. NZ Med J 1993; 106:531 (Letter).
69. Lawrie SM, Pelosi AJ. Chronic fatigue syndrome and myalgic encephalomyelitis. Br Med J 1994; 309:275 (Letter).
70. Simpson LO. Myalgic encephalomyelitis and chronic fatigue syndrome. NZ Med J 1995:108:44-5 (Letter).
71. Bates DW, Buchwald D, Lee J. et al. A comparison of case definitions of chronic fatigue syndrome. Clin Infect Dis 1994:18 (Suppl 1):S11-5.
72. Fukuda K, Strauss SE, Hickie I, et al. The chronic fatigue syndrome: a comprehensive approach to its definition and study. International Chronic Fatigue Syndrome Study Group. Ann Intern Med 1994; 121:953-9.
73. Dodge JA, Kim MW. The chronic fatigue syndrome. Ann Intern Med 1995; 123:75 (letter).

74. Scott S, Deary I, Pelosi AJ. General practitioners' attitudes to patients with as self-diagnosis of myalgic encephalomyelitis. Br Med J 1995; 310:508.
75. Hurel SJ, Abuiasha B, Baylis PH, et al. Patients with a self-diagnosis of myalgic encephalomyelitis. Br Med J 1995; 311:329 (Letter).
76. Arber M. GP's attitudes to a self-diagnosis of myalgic encephalomyelitis. Sufferers continue to be misrepresented. Br Med J 1995; 310:1330 (Letter).
77. Shepherd C. GP's attitudes to a self-diagnosis of ME. Evidence supports the presence of encephalitis. Br Med J 1995; 310:1330 (Letter).
78. Sutton GC. 'Too tired to go to the support group': a health needs assessment of myalgic encephalomyelitis. J Pub Health Med 1996; 18:343-9.
79. Simpson LO. Myalgic encephalomyelitis (ME): a haemorheological disorder manifested as impaired capillary blood flow. J Orthomol Med 1997; 12:69-76.
80. Simpson LO, Herbison GP. The results from red cell shape analyses of blood samples from members of myalgic encephalomyelitis organisations in 4 countries. J Orthomol Med 1997; 12:221-6.
81. Marshall EP, Williams M, Hooper M. What is ME? What is CFS? Information for clinicians and lawyers. December 2001.
82. Simpson LO. On the pathophysiology of ME/CFS. NZ Fam Physn 2002; 29:426-8.
83. Simpson LO, O'Neill DJ. Red cell shape changes in the blood of people 60 years of age and older imply a role for blood rheology in the aging process. Gerontology 2003; 49:310-6.
84. Puri BK. Long chain polyunsaturated fatty acids and the pathophysiology of myalgic encephalomyelitis (chronic fatigue syndrome). J Clin Pathol 2007; 60:122-4
85. Carruthers BM. Definitions and aetiology of myalgic encephalomyelitis: how the Canadian consensus of myalgic encephalomyelitis works. J Clin Pathol 2007; 60:117-9.
86. Hyde BM. The Nightingale Myalgic Encephalomyelitis (M.E.) Definition. The Nightingale Research Foundation, Ottawa, Canada, 2007.
87. Dormehl IC, Jordaan B, Oliver DW, et al. SPECT monitoring of improved cerebral blood flow during long-term treatment of elderly patients with nootropic drugs. Clin Nucl Med 1999; 24:29-34.

CHAPTER IV
- THE POST-ME ERA

The main objective in dealing with this topic is to provide ME sufferers with some idea of the various concepts and opinions which continue to oppose the recognition of ME as a clinical entity with its own requirements for management and treatment. It would seem that in this era there has been a vast expenditure of time and money into various aspects of chronic illnesses but with little apparent benefit to those who suffer from ME. A search for "Chronic fatigue syndrome in English," in the PubMed search engine produced 3054 titles, so it should be noted that there is no intention to undertake an exhaustive analysis of the published literature. Instead, the objective will be to examine the various trends and fashions which share the common feature of diverging from ME.

CFS Working Case Definitions, 1988 – 1996

It would seem appropriate to consider that the beginning of this Era was marked by the release from the Centres of Disease Control of a working case definition of chronic fatigue syndrome (CFS), which was constructed primarily for research purposes (1). Apparently, in order to justify the term "chronic," the disorder had to be severe enough to reduce daily activity by at least 50% for more than six months.

> Appropriate treatment for ME should include a prescription for rest immediately upon becoming ill. Implicit in this (CDC) definition is that the patient must wait six months for a diagnosis, yet according to very early reports, the prognosis for level and duration of disability depends upon the patient's ability to rest during the first six months.

The key factor was a persisting or relapsing fatigue, or easy fatigability which was not alleviated by bed rest. In addition, the diagnosis required the presence of some minor criteria and the exclusion of other chronic conditions, including chronic psychiatric illness. Thus, in order to satisfy the CDC criteria, patients were required to exhibit both major criteria and either eight minor or six minor and two physical criteria. Although the easy fatigability was in accord with Ramsay's concept, there is no recognition of the remissions which are a feature of ME. While the discrepancies between the two concepts are so great that they clearly do not refer to the same condition, **the CFS criteria are so encompassing that they could incorporate ME.** An early response to the introduction of CFS was a reduction in the use of the label 'ME', which was replaced by 'CFS' or by 'ME/CFS'.

Some semantic/linguistic subtleties are going on here: **Replacement** of one term by another suggests a **complete overlap** of the condition referred to – **the same entity by another name**. The category **ME/CFS** introduces the possibility that there are **two different and separate conditions** which are both being referred to or the possibility that **ME may be a condition which includes the sub-group, CFS**. In the UK today, what you will find is **CFS/ME**, which again raises the possibility that **two distinct conditions** are being referred to, or that **perhaps they are one and the same, or perhaps that ME is a subcategory of CFS**. These apparently minor distinctions will have an effect on how we think about the entities so labelled. This effect will be reinforced by **the direction of the shift**: ME to CFS, ME/CFS, CFS/ME subtly moves ME from existing in its own right, towards becoming a category subsumed by and within the category CFS. Then the widening category 'CFS' (widened in the UK by the Oxford criteria, **which don't even include the damaging effects of exercise and yet are a central feature in most descriptions of ME**) begins to open up the possibility first, of **including psychiatric conditions** that are also characterised by fatigue, second, of movement towards **labelling the entire larger category as a form of psychiatric problem, and including ME within it.**

And, of course, an important effect of such imprecise labelling is that meaningful research becomes impossible without a clear definition of what it is that one is researching, and a clear specification of what symptoms a person has to present with to be included in the cohort being researched.

Hooper discusses this process in detail in his article 'Magical Medicine – How to Make A Disease Disappear' [11]

The rest of this section illustrates in detail the progress and effects of this process of widening definitions and the inclusion of more and more psychiatric conditions within them. In regard to fatigue connected to depression, it is notable that **the important distinction between the physical tiredness of ME and the lack of motivation characteristic of depression is never made. Not wanting to do anything** is not the same thing as **becoming exhausted from minimal physical exertion**, and recognising and acknowledging that would make a differential diagnosis between ME and depression very straightforward.

It is of interest that prior to the release of the CDC working case definition, an American group (2) discussed the role of Epstein-Barr virus in persisting illness and fatigue. The authors stated

> *Twenty-five young or middle-aged adults presented with a chronic but relatively stable fatiguing illness. The group is somewhat homogeneous in the nature and degree of constitutional complaints and the apparent lack of substantial physical findings or abnormalities in routine laboratory tests. An important feature of the patient group was a degree of disability, seemingly out of proportion to the objective extent of the illness.*

Three years later, an English group made similar observations about Coxsackie B2 virus (3) which led to the suggestion that, *"...a persistent viral infection has an aetiological role."* It was concluded

However, it is likely that although enteroviruses are major aetiological agents of Postviral Fatigue Syndrome, other viruses, particularly Epstein-Barr virus, may induce the syndrome. We suggest that this disease is a chronic metabolic myopathy induced by persistent viral infection.

But as the results from ninety-six muscle biopsies showed that only twenty were positive for enterovirus-specific RNA, the suggestion was not sustainable.

The CDC working case definition soon came under critical scrutiny. Manu et al (4) noted "The frequency of the chronic fatigue syndrome in medical practice is not known. We applied the criteria of a recent consensus definition to one hundred thirty-five patients evaluated in a clinic for chronic fatigue." The panel comprised fifty-three men and eighty-two women who had suffered from debilitating fatigue for six months or more, and the authors reported

Only six patients fulfilled the criteria for this diagnosis (CFS). Moreover, two of these six patients were diagnosed within six months as having somatization disorder and one patient developed neurologic abnormalities highly suspicious of multiple sclerosis and one patient showed considerable improvement after taking antidepressant drugs. Thus it appears that the chronic fatigue syndrome, as defined, is uncommon, even among patients with chronic fatigue and rare if the patients are carefully evaluated and followed up.

Possibly as an indication of dissatisfaction with the CDC case definition, other guidelines were set out in a letter to Lancet, from an Australian group, (5) which drew an objection from Ramsay (6) to the claim that the term, "myalgic encephalomyelitis" was inappropriate. In contrast to Ramsay's complaint, the staff of the Institute of Psychiatry (7) stated, "*Dr. Lloyd and colleagues are to be commended for considering the case definition of chronic fatigue syndrome.*" The Australian guidelines were used in a study of the prevalence of CFS in an Australian community (8) but as it involved only a small number of cases, the results should be treated with caution.

Staff from the Institute of Psychiatry published the "Oxford" guidelines, the following year. (9) Both the Australian and Oxford guidelines agreed with the CDC case definition in regard to the six month's duration; that there was functional impairment, and that known physical causes could be a basis for exclusion. However, both guidelines differed from the CDC concept in terms of the presence of cognitive and neuropsychiatric symptoms, and there were minor differences in the lists of psychiatric exclusions.

Perhaps the first recognition that CFS encompassed a heterogeneous population was noted in a paper by Krupp et al (10) which stated

The 1988 definition of CFS by the Centres for Disease Control encompasses several conditions in which the major characteristic is severe fatigue, associated with constitutional symptoms.

The authors concluded

CFS appears to be a heterogeneous entity. Although there may be a high coincidence of major depression in CFS, a substantial proportion of patients lack

any DSM-III-R psychiatric disorder, yet still manifest the syndrome, thereby suggesting that it has an autonomous entity. Despite the evolving nature of our current understanding of CFS, a rational diagnostic and therapeutic approach to CFS is possible.

Unfortunately, that optimism appears to be ill-founded, and a contrary viewpoint was expressed by Lane et al (11) after evaluating two hundred adult patients with a chief complaint of chronic fatigue. They found that patients who met the criteria for CFS did not differ from fatigued control subjects in terms of current psychiatric disorders, active mood disorders and pre-existing psychiatric disorders. It was concluded *"Patients with CFS have a high prevalence of unrecognised, current psychiatric disorders, which often predate their fatigue syndrome."* In a later paper from the same group (12) which reported similar findings, it was noted

We conclude that most patients with a chief complaint of chronic fatigue, including those exhibiting the features of CFS, suffer from standard mood, anxiety and/or somatoform disorders. Careful research is still needed to determine whether CFS is a distinct entity or a variant of these psychiatric illnesses.

In a report of the proceedings of a workshop on CFS at the NIH in March 1991, (13) it was recommended that the CDC case definition be modified, *"...to exclude fewer patients from analyses because of a history of psychiatric disorder."* Consistent with the views expressed by Krupp et al (10) it was stated, *"Because CFS is not a homogeneous abnormality and because there is no single pathogenic mechanism, research progress may depend upon delineation of these and other patient sub-groups for separate data analysis."* A similar view was expressed by Levine, (14) who noted that because some investigators preferred CFS to ME, *"...it is quite likely that we are discussing a multiplicity of entities."*

Albany N.Y. was the venue for international conferences on clinical aspects of CFIDS/ME on October 2 and 3, and a research conference on CFS/ME on October 3 and 4, 1992. Although many of the speakers at the CFIDS meeting did not provide abstracts for the programme there were several interesting contributions. Dr. Hyde provided a historical perspective of CFIDS, and he concluded

The concept of 'Chronic Fatigue' has unintentionally created considerable disparagement of patients ill with this post-infectious disease process. CFS is an inappropriate name and should be abandoned.

In a section titled, "The immune system: friend or foe," Dr. Andrew Lloyd stated "Nevertheless, current data do provide circumstantial support for the hypothesis that CFS results from an altered immune response to an immunological challenge." This proposal was challenged by Dr. Komaroff, who, even though he was speaking at a CFIDS meeting, concluded

CFS seems likely to have a multifactorial etiology, like most illnesses. While the discovery of a single explanation, such as a novel infectious agent or a specific inherited immunological defect, might simplify the search for solutions to this illness, we are dubious that such a simple answer will emerge.

But if the multifactorial causes had the same effect of changing the internal environment and inducing change in red cell shape populations and reduced red cell deformability, then maybe the 'simple answer' to the search for a solution could be impaired capillary blood flow.

Speaking on the topic of CFS in adults and children, Dr. David Bell stated "Adolescents and adults share the same symptom pattern of CFIDS. However, children who develop CFIDS prior to puberty usually have a gradual onset of symptoms in contrast to the acute onset of older children." Dr. Sandman concluded his contribution on "CFIDS and depression" by stating "…depression is not irrevocably related to CFIDS, although they can co-exist."

But, as noted by Mena et al, concerning the results from SPECT scans, "These findings suggest that there is diminution of cerebral blood flow in both conditions (CFS and late life depression), etc."

As there are several other reports with similar findings of reduced regional cerebral blood flow in depression, such findings imply that inadequate supplies of oxygen and nutrient substrates could be a causal factor in depressive illness.

In addressing the topic, "Biological response modifier therapy" Dr. Peterson drew attention to the variable success rate of proposed therapies and concluded, "*Methodological problems in CFIDS studies are abundant.*"

However, the most intriguing contribution was by Dr. J. H. Renner, titled "Conceptions and misconceptions about chronic fatigue syndrome," and as the message is still relevant today his abstract is reproduced here, verbatim:

Publicity about chronic fatigue syndrome – CFS – has been very confusing to patients, physicians, researchers, the media, governmental agencies, insurance companies and employers. Numerous 'breakthrough' research announcements about CFS have occurred with regularity. These announcements make headlines but are seldom confirmed or verified by any other scientists. Patients with CFS confront their physicians with tidbits of information about diagnostic ideas and therapeutic treatments which a cautious physician rightly questions and thereby will await scientific verification before jumping to conclusions. Many examples of both media mistakes and premature conclusions from questionable research will be presented. Solid, peer-reviewed research reported at scientific meetings and published in peer-reviewed journals is one solution to the serious dilemma over credibility. Research misconduct and questionable research practices are not the same thing. There will be some discussion of possible harm to the public from misconduct in research. Material will be presented from RESPONSIBLE SCIENCE, ensuring the integrity of the research process, by the National Academy of Sciences. Some physicians see advertisements in newspapers about an entrepreneurially oriented physician treating a thousand CFS patients and 'curing' them. These physicians ask, 'What is going on?' They wonder how many patients are there really with CFS. What is this so-called 'cure'? Another reason – and often an over-riding one – that there are so many sceptics about CFS, is the frequent occurrence of medical and economic abuse that physicians have seen perpetrated on patients diagnosed with this difficult medical problem. Sixty different treatments have been recorded. Some are obviously inappropriate.

It should be obvious that the points which Dr. Renner makes about CFS are just as relevant to ME.

In contrast to the CFIDS programme, all the speakers at the CFS/ME Research Conference provided abstracts. While the programme was very diversified, there was little new or important information. Even though there are recognised problems concerning case definitions, there were some epidemiological studies presented. While some studies have concluded that cases meeting the case definition of CFS are uncommon, this seemed to be confirmed in one study and challenged by another. One study noted the prevalence of CFS in Atlanta as 1.8 per 100,000; 3.8 in Grand Rapids; 4.4 in Wichita and 6.0 in Reno. But in a questionnaire-based study of 1474 nurses, a prevalence of 380 per 100,000 was claimed.

Topics in the general field of immunology were the most frequently discussed – although the relevance was not always clear. One study showed that minorities with CFS had higher values for six different, inexpensive measures of immune function, but as only 20% to about 30% were involved, this raises questions about the significance of the tests. The results were interpreted as suggesting "*…chronic low level activation of the immune system in CFS.*" Another investigation into immunological abnormalities found a marked decrease in natural killer cell activity "*…in almost all CFS patients involved*" but how the finding related to the fatigue state was not discussed. The possible involvement of the immune system in CFS was not made clearer by a study of soluble immune mediators. It was concluded "*The results summarised above indicate that CFS is associated with imbalance in the levels of soluble immune mediators, which in turn are linked to CD8+ T cell activation.*" However, is an "association" a pathogenic factor?

Although an in vitro study of Ampligen showed the drug to be "*…a potent inhibitor of HHV-6 replication*" this finding seemed not to be transferable to a clinical trial, where forty-five CFS patients were given the drug by twice-weekly IV infusions. Over 90% of patients completed the twenty-four weeks of treatment. In contrast to the in vitro study of HHV-6, it was stated, "*The subjects in this study had many objective abnormalities suggesting virologic/immunologic involvement in their disease process.*" However, as no viral presence was identified, it is unclear how they could conclude that the treatment had beneficial effects.

I presented our study of the effects of trigger-finger fatigue on red cell shape just prior to lunch on the second day of the meeting. During the lunch break, I was asked if I would meet with patients after the conclusion of the meeting. I was pleased with the invitation and notices went up advising patients to meet with Dr. Simpson at 4.30pm. More than twenty people from different parts of the USA came to the meeting and were soon involved in a vigorous discussion about the pros and cons of CFS vs. ME. Time passed very quickly and at 6pm a janitor arrived and asked that the room be vacated. The patients left in small groups still engaged in discussion.

As had been arranged previously, a manuscript dealing with the study was submitted to the Journal of Infectious Diseases, but the paper was rejected with the request that it be re-written. Evidently **the editor did not accept that red cells came in different shape classes,** as after the third revision was rejected, I withdrew the paper. I do not know how many other papers were rejected, but in the proceedings of the meeting there is no record of my presentation. Eventually the paper was published in the New Zealand Medical Journal.

> So here is another example of a supposedly objective scientist rejecting evidence that is before his eyes in the form of micrographs of red blood cells having varying shapes, in favour, apparently, of accepting the dogma that 'all red blood cells are biconcave discocytes', end of story. Again, doctors refuse to entertain anything which is outside their taught parameters, and, again, patients are thereby deprived of information that could improve their well-being.

During a search for the prevalence of unusual debilitating fatigue and its relationship to CFS or other illnesses, one thousand consecutive patients attending an outpatient clinic were screened (15). Five patients were excluded because of a previous diagnosis of CFS, and the results showed that eighty-five of nine hundred ninety-five patients had an unexplained, debilitating fatigue which had persisted for at least six months. As forty-eight patients declined further evaluation, and eleven were lost to follow up, only twenty-six were evaluated. After three cases with hypothyroidism and one case with a major psychiatric disorder were removed, it was found that of the remaining twenty-two cases, three met the CDC criteria; four met the British criteria and ten met the Australian case definition. The authors concluded, *"While chronic, debilitating fatigue is common in medical outpatients, CFS is relatively uncommon. Prevalence depends substantially on the case definition used."*

Subsequently, the same group (16) compared how the three case definitions related to eight hundred and five patients from two institutions. They reported that 61% met the CDC criteria; 56% met the Australian criteria, and 55% met the British criteria. The proportions were relatively similar for patients from both institutions. It was concluded *"These data suggest that the more inclusive case definitions may be superior."* That conclusion was reflected in a revision of the CDC guidelines with more inclusive criteria, (17) which included a *"…strategy for sub-grouping fatigued persons in formal investigations."* While other authors had proposed the need to sub-classify CFS patients, the proposal seemed to formalise the earlier proposal by Levine (14) that *"One useful aspect of international working groups could be the development of improved guidelines to sub-classify CFS using sub-groups such as those with or without documented immune dysfunction, etc."*

But if there is a need to sub-group CFS patients, then this does raise serious questions about the logic and validity of the CDC guidelines. **Is there any real value in grouping patients with similar symptoms which could be manifestations of disparate disorders with different aetiologies?** The fact that sub-grouping is recommended to understand better the nature of CFS draws attention to the major problem in the field – the lack of an agreed pathophysiology.

In a study of the prevalence of CFS, (18) four thousand randomly selected subjects attending a health maintenance organisation were evaluated by questionnaire which achieved a 77% response rate. Of the five hundred and ninety responders who suffered from chronic fatigue, the fatigue of three hundred and eighty-eight could be accounted for by an existing medical or psychiatric condition. Of the seventy-four persons who had unexplained chronic fatigue, only three met the CDC criteria for CFS. This low incidence of three cases of CFS in five hundred and eighty people who suffered from chronic fatigue seemed not to be reflected in the conclusions which stated

> *Using different assumptions about the likelihood that persons who did not participate in the study had the chronic fatigue syndrome, the estimated crude point prevalence of the syndrome in this community ranged from seventy-five to two-hundred and sixty-seven cases per one hundred thousand persons. The point prevalence of chronic fatigue alone was strikingly higher; it ranged from one thousand seven hundred and seventy-five to six thousand three hundred and twenty-one cases per one hundred thousand persons.*

A similar study from the Wessely School in England, (19) concerned questionnaire measures of fatigue and psychological symptoms and one thousand nine hundred and eighty-five subjects responded. Six months later, two hundred and fourteen subjects with chronic fatigue were compared with two hundred and fourteen matched subjects without fatigue in terms of a number of variables. The results showed that whether they were assessed by questionnaire or interview, those suffering from chronic fatigue were more likely to be at greater risk for current psychiatric disorder than non-fatigued subjects, and this was true also for those suffering from CFS. However it was noted that three symptoms (post-exertion malaise, muscle weakness and myalgia) occurred more frequently in CFS patients. The authors reached the controversial, but probably predictable conclusion that

> *Most subjects with chronic fatigue or chronic fatigue syndrome in primary care also meet criteria for a current psychiatric disorder. Both chronic fatigue and chronic fatigue syndrome are associated with previous psychiatric disorder, partly explained by high rates of current psychiatric disorder. The symptoms thought to represent a specific process in chronic fatigue syndrome may be related to the joint experience of somatic and psychological distress.*

This conclusion highlights the difference between CFS and ME in terms of Ramsay's criteria, where the existence of a psychiatric disorder would exclude a diagnosis of ME.

Working in the same general field, an American group reported on the results of a study in which a group of three hundred and sixty-nine patients with debilitating fatigue included two hundred and eighty-one cases who met the major criteria of the CDC case definition but without evidence of organic or psychiatric illness (20). In addition 91% of cases also met the minor criteria. The relevant clinical and laboratory data were contrasted with those from three hundred and eleven healthy control subjects and from two "comparison" groups; viz, twenty-five subjects with relapsing–remitting multiple sclerosis and nineteen cases of major depression. It was concluded that

Patients meeting the major criteria of the current working case definition of CFS reported symptoms which were clearly distinguishable from the experience of healthy control subjects and from disease comparison groups with multiple sclerosis and depression.

The fact that multiple sclerosis and major depression were chosen as comparison groups deserves special scrutiny.

Possible Aetiological Similarities
CFS, multiple sclerosis, depression

Although Komaroff et al (20) provided no reasons for selecting multiple sclerosis and depression as their "comparison groups", it is of considerable interest that altered blood flow is a significant factor in both disorders. In addition, the symptoms of MS include the following; blurred or double vision, problems with walking, balance and co-ordination, stiffness and spasm, numbness and 'pins and needles', shakiness, speech difficulties, poor memory and difficulty in thinking logically, painful muscle spasms, fatigue, muscle weakness, difficulties in swallowing and erectile dysfunction in men. It is noteworthy that many of these symptoms are also problems in CFS patients. In order to provide a better perspective, the evidence of blood flow problems and altered blood rheology in MS and depression will be reviewed.

(a) Multiple sclerosis

After the publication of our 1986 study which showed that ME blood filtered poorly, we were alerted to the fact that persistent tiredness was also a problem of people with MS. In an ethically approved study, we investigated several features of blood samples obtained from three male and twelve female outpatient volunteers with clinically definite MS. Control data were obtained from twenty-five male and twenty-five female blood donors of similar ages to the MS people. (21)

Just as in the ME study, it was found that MS blood filtered poorly in comparison with blood donor blood. In addition, whole blood viscosity of MS females was higher than that of controls at three different shear rates, but in MS males the increase in blood viscosity was notable only at low shear rate. Differences were found in red cell membrane fatty acids with MS red cells having less sphingomyelin but more phosphate-idylinositol plus phosphatidylserine than control red cells. Scanning electron microscopy of red blood cells showed that MS red cells had different shapes from that of control red cells. Thus this small study indicated that MS blood rheology was abnormal.

Therefore it is relevant that several early papers considered that problems of blood flow played a role in the formation of plaques in the brain. In a 1958 paper describing subcutaneous haemorrhages in MS patients, Swank (22) stated that "...*the vascular system and especially the blood itself*" were involved in the pathogenesis of MS. Twenty five years later he published a report which showed with the use of Xenon 133, that the rate of cerebral blood flow and red cell delivery in MS patients was much less than in non-MS controls. (23)

It seems noteworthy that the situation in MS patients, where shape-changed red cells were associated with impaired cerebral blood flow, seems to reproduce the situation in ME patients who also have shape-changed red cells, and reduced rates of regional cerebral blood flow have been demonstrated by SPECT scans.

Such observations stimulated a study of the haematology and red cell shape in MS people. After obtaining ethical committee approval for the study, which was funded in part by the New Zealand Multiple Sclerosis Society, letters were sent to MS societies, four in the South Island and two in the North Island, outlining the features of the proposed study and seeking the co-operation of their members. After receiving notice of their interest, the societies were requested to arrange dates and venues for the collection of blood samples. At the pre-arranged times, I used a slide sequence to explain to patients and their relatives the aims and objectives of the study. Following a question and answer session, volunteers signed consent forms and completed a simple questionnaire which requested details of their age and the age at which MS was diagnosed and details of their mobility, medication and symptoms. Blood samples were obtained from one hundred and sixty-six women aged between twenty-four and seventy-four years and fifty-four men aged between twenty-six and seventy-one years. Similar percentages of both sexes (58% women, 53% men) could walk without the use of a walking aid.

Blood samples were obtained from an ante-cubital vein by experienced venepuncturists, after the cuff had been released to ensure that the sample came from flowing blood. Within seconds of the needle being withdrawn from the vein, three drops of blood were mixed with 5ml of fixative and eventually processed for scanning electron microscopy. The remainder of the blood sample was anti-coagulated with EDTA for an automated blood screen. Having determined that no changes in blood samples which had been treated similarly occurred in the first twenty-four hours, arrangements were made to courier blood samples to Dunedin where they were screened on the same H6000 Technicon haematology auto-analyser. As a result of such arrangements, all blood samples were screened within twenty hours of the sample being drawn. Control blood samples were obtained from blood donors and healthy volunteers, and involved twenty-nine men aged between twenty-two and seventy years and twenty-three women aged between nineteen and sixty years.

The haematology data showed that 18.5% of MS men and 14% of women had haematocrits which were higher than the upper limits of the reference ranges. In addition 25.9% of men and 18.7% of women had total leucocyte values which were above the reference ranges. Red cell shape analysis showed that MS blood samples had abnormally high values for cells with surface changes and for early cup forms. An interesting but unexplained observation was that linear regression showed a significant relationship between total leucocyte count and latitude, with the lowest counts in the south and the highest in the north.

With the aim of seeking more information about this finding, application was made to the New Zealand Multiple Sclerosis Society for funds to study blood samples from MS people living in the northern cities. In response, the Society stated that the Medical Advisory Committee had advised that no further funding should be provided to Dr. Simpson until he had validated his technique. The validation involved the analysis of sixty blinded blood samples provided by the committee, and I agreed immediately.

During the time we awaited the arrival of the validating samples, we embarked on an ethical-committee approved study of the effects of evening primrose oil on the symptoms of MS people. The study was based upon the fact that the gammalinolenic acid in the primrose oil would raise the blood levels of prostaglandin E1. A 1974 study (24) had used spin-labelled erythrocytes to show that prostaglandin E1 made erythrocytes more deformable. That finding was confirmed in the following year (25) when it was reported that prostaglandin E1 increased the rate of filtration through a standard filter. We obtained similar results in a small study which showed that 4.5 grams daily of evening primrose oil increased the filterability of the blood from cigarette smokers. So the expectation was that if MS symptoms reflected the adverse effects of poorly deformable red cells, then a daily intake of nine x 500mg capsules of evening primrose oil should provide symptomatic relief.

On the receipt of a signed consent form, participants were provided with sufficient oil capsules for twelve weeks at a daily intake of nine capsules. One half of the panel were provided with evening primrose oil, the other half received capsules identical in appearance but containing safflower oil. At the conclusion of the twelve week supplementation period, participants were requested to complete a simple questionnaire which sought information on two points. During the twelve weeks of the study, did your symptoms get worse, stay the same or get better? Tick one selection. If your symptoms got worse, list in order of severity, the nature of those symptoms. If your symptoms got better, list in order of benefit, the names of the symptoms which improved.

The responses showed that those subjects taking evening primrose oil had improved in all sorts of ways, which ranged from a general improvement in quality of life to relief from constipation. Several days after the conclusion of the study, a man who had been taking evening primrose oil, but had reported that his symptoms stayed the same, came into the office to report that a few days after he had mailed the questionnaire, he had noticed problems with his vision, and he wanted to change his questionnaire response.

However, I was unable to find a neurology journal which was willing to publish the findings concerning red cell shape and haematology in MS people. As there is little published information concerning haematology in MS, I attempted to obtain an estimate by asking one hundred and twenty-two MS people how frequently they had had a blood test in the range, regularly, occasionally, seldom and never. Occasional blood tests were reported by 21%; 39% seldom had blood tests and 29% had never had a blood test. The 10% of cases who had regular blood tests reported that they were tests relating to thyroid function or to warfarin. Because the primary study was not published, there seemed to be little logic in preparing the evening primrose oil study for publication.

About two years after the validation study was initiated, instead of the expected 60 blood samples, 28 samples were received from the Medical Advisory Committee of the Multiple Sclerosis Society. The samples were duly processed and the results returned to the Advisory

LESLIE O. SIMPSON & NANCY BLAKE

Committee, which sent the details of the MS and non-MS neurological disorders. Analysis of the data by a biostatistician showed that despite the smallness of the numbers, the MS blood samples were highly significantly different from the non-MS samples. A letter published in the New Zealand Medical Journal, titled, "Red cell shape in multiple sclerosis," (26) is the only outcome of more than four years work.

It seems reasonable to conclude that the blood flow problems resulting from altered blood rheology contribute to the lifestyle difficulties faced by MS people.

(b) Depressive illness

No information about red cell shape in depression is available as I never obtained the co-operation of psychologists or psychiatrists which was necessary to obtain blood samples. While the relevance of the information is uncertain, blood samples provided by a small number of patients with bipolar disorder showed shape-changed red cell populations.

The role of blood flow in depressive illness will be considered in terms of studies involving different neuroimaging techniques. An American group used Xenon inhalation; an English group used positron emission tomography (PET); various groups used single photon emission computed tomography (SPECT), to study cerebral blood flow in depression.

Sackeim et al published the results of five studies under the general title, "Regional cerebral blood flow in mood disorders," all of which were based upon the use of Xenon inhalation to measure regional cerebral blood flow (rCBF).

The first study was "Comparison of major depressives and normal controls at rest", (27) in which the authors stated "Since excitation and inhibition are energy-dependent processes, biochemical derangements should result in abnormalities in regional cerebral blood flow, etc." Yet if blood flow was impaired, but not as a result of a "biochemical derangement", the resulting reduction in rates of delivery of oxygen and nutrient substrates would inhibit biochemical activity. This apparently back-to-front concept was repeated in different terms: "Consistent patterns of alteration of cerebral blood flow and cerebral metabolic rate in discrete functional brain systems may result (my underlining) from a variety of neurochemical processes." But it is difficult to imagine how normal biochemical activity could proceed if the rate of blood flow reached sub-normal levels. However, it is rare for biochemical concepts to include recognition of the fact that in many conditions the rates of capillary blood flow may be sub-normal.

The interpretation of the results would have been made difficult by the age factor in the make-up of the study panel. On the basis of the information provided, the 95% confidence intervals for the ages of males was 36.8 to 83.8 years and for females it was 34.3 to 86.4 years. In 1992 it would not have been known that after about 55 years, the aging process is associated with increased blood viscosity and changed shape populations of red cells. Therefore the proportion of participants over 55 years of age would influence any assessment of blood flow, and for that reason it was not surprising that the results showed, "...that an elderly sample of patients with major depressive disorder had both a global flow

RAMSAY'S DISEASE - ME

deficit and an abnormal distribution." Global blood flow in those with depression was about 12% lower than in controls. The authors stated

> *In psychiatric disorders, cerebral blood flow is typically assessed as an indirect means of measuring the integrity of cerebral metabolism. Flow and glucose metabolism in the normal brain are tightly coupled on a local basis. ……Therefore, the global and regional abnormalities we observed in cerebral blood flow most likely indicate metabolic abnormalities.*

While it was stated *"The cause of the rCBF deficits is unknown"*, the problem was considered only from the viewpoint of vascular change.

The second study in the series was titled "Comparison of major depression and Alzheimer's disease" (28) which reached the expected conclusion that 30 patients with major depression and 30 patients with Alzheimer's disease had, *"…markedly reduced global cortical blood flow."*

The third study, "Treatment and clinical response," (29) described the assessment of cortical blood flow by the Xenon 133 technique, prior to and after electroconvulsive therapy. According to the results, the treatment did not reverse the cerebral blood flow abnormalities of major depression. But, rather surprisingly, it was noted that in the acute period, blood flow reduction *"…both globally and in particular patterns of brain regions, were associated with a superior clinical outcome following the treatment course."* It is not easy to understand how reducing the rate of blood flow in depression could lead to "a superior clinical outcome," when it had previously been noted that cerebral metabolic abnormalities were associated with reduced blood flow rates. The authors concluded *"The therapeutic properties of electroconvulsive therapy are related to a reduced functional brain activity in specific neural regions."* But it remains unexplained why the clinical outcome was better when the blood flow abnormalities were not different from those which were present in the depressed state.

"Comparison of mania and depression" was the title of the fourth study (30), which reported that in the resting state, there were significant reductions in rCBF in the anterior cortical areas of patients in both the manic and the depressed groups. Apart from differences in the rCBF localised to the inferior frontal cortex, between clinical groups, it was concluded *"The evidence in this study suggests that young adult manic and depressed patients are predominantly similar in cortical rCBF parameters."* How this conclusion might relate to the findings of the effects of electroconvulsive therapy was not discussed. Nor do the findings provide a basis for understanding the pathophysiology of mania unless manic changes involved other regions of the brain.

In 2001, the fifth paper in the series was published, under the title "Effects of antidepressant medication in late-life depression" (31) which reported the assessment of rCBF by Xenon inhalation, after nine weeks of treatment with one of two antidepressants, in twenty elderly patients with late-life depression (who on the basis of current knowledge would have altered blood rheology). Those who responded to treatment showed reduced perfusion in the frontal regions of the brain. The report concluded *"These findings are consistent with this group's previous report of reduced rCBF after response to*

139

LESLIE O. SIMPSON & NANCY BLAKE

electroconvulsive therapy, and suggest a common mechanism of action." However, because of the physical nature of blood (it is a thixotropic system) a reduction in flow rate would lead to an increase in blood viscosity, adding further resistance to flow. The persistence with which improved function is associated with reduced rCBF is puzzling, as the baseline data showed reduced perfusion of the frontal cortical region, but this situation was not changed by those who responded to antidepressants.

It will be of interest to find what other techniques reveal.

In contrast to the use of Xenon inhalation to assess cerebral blood flow, positron emission tomography (PET) was used by an English group in several studies of patients with depressive illness. In 1992, this group published a paper titled "The anatomy of melancholia – focal abnormalities of cerebral blood flow in major depression" (32) which reported the use of PET to measure regional cerebral blood flow (rCBF) in thirty-three patients with primary depression. Ten of the patients also had "*an associated, severe, cognitive impairment.*" As a whole, the depressed patients had decreased rCBF in two regions of the brain, while in those with cognitive impairment there was decreased blood flow in another region (left medial frontal gyrus), but an increase in rCBF in another region (the cerebellar vermis). The authors concluded "*Therefore an anatomical dissociation has been described between depressed mood and depression-related cognitive impairment.*"

A year later (33) they reported similar findings in a larger group of patients and concluded "*These data indicate that symptomatic specificity may be ascribed to regional functional deficits in major depressive illness.*" (It is very relevant, that in 1997, Lucey et al (34) reported that different patterns of cerebral blood flow had been found in patients suffering from obsessive compulsive disorder, panic disorder with agoraphobia and post-traumatic stress disorder.)

The English group continued to explore the relationship between rCBF, as assessed by PET, and neuropsychological dysfunction in depression. (35) Their conclusion that "*The findings provide additional evidence that the neuropsychological deficits in depression are associated with abnormalities in regional brain function, and in particular with the function of the medial prefrontal cortex*" fits very well with my beliefs concerning brain dysfunction in ME.

That conclusion was mirrored in the findings of another report which concerned rCBF in depression and how it related to clinical observations. (36) After an examination of the relationships between depressive symptoms and patterns of rCBF it was concluded "*These data indicate that symptomatic specificity may be ascribed to regional functional deficits in major depressive illnesses.*"

However, in terms of the importance of normal blood flow to sustain normal brain function, their study of the changes in rCBF on recovery from depression is of some significance.(37) Twenty five of the forty patients who had been scanned previously were re-scanned following clinical remission. The authors stated

> *The previously described relationship between clinical symptoms and brain perfusion in the depressed state was no longer present in the recovered state; this supports the hypothesis of state relatedness. Thus, recovery from depression is*

140

associated with increases in rCBF in the same areas in which focal decreases are described in the depressed state, in comparison with normal controls.

This demonstration of an association of dysfunction associated with reduced rCBF highlights the problems of the American concept, based upon Xenon inhalation, that reduced rCBF was associated with a "superior clinical outcome."

Single photon emission computed tomography (SPECT) is another technique for assessing blood flow, and in a 1991 paper, O'Connell et al (38) stated *"…it was of use in the diagnosis of medically ill patients who also presented with psychopathology…..Often changes in regional cerebral blood flow are seen before structural changes become apparent on CT or MRI."*

An Edinburgh group (39) used SPECT to study, at rest, forty patients with a major depressive episode. Their technique involved the intra-venous injection of a ligand (99mTc-exametazine) to provide an estimate of brain metabolism, as it was taken up in the brain in proportion to rCBF. The authors stated *"The depressed group showed reduced uptake (i.e. reduced rCBF) in the majority of cortical and sub-cortical regions examined, most significantly in temporal, inferior frontal and parietal areas."*

A group of American workers (which included Dr. Komaroff, who had previously used multiple sclerosis and depression as "comparison groups," in a CFS study) compared brain SPECT scans from patients with CFS, AIDS dementia complex and major unipolar depression (40). A special analysis of variance was used to analyse the data related to "regional defects" and "mid-cerebral uptake indexes." As people with AIDS have been shown to have altered red cell shape populations, this could be a factor in the analysis which showed that the highest number of defects occurred in patients with AIDS dementia complex, and *"Patients with chronic fatigue syndrome and depression had similar numbers of defects per patient."* In all groups, defects were mainly in the frontal and temporal lobes. It is unclear how the authors were able to conclude

These findings are consistent with the hypothesis that chronic fatigue syndrome may be due to chronic viral encephalitis; clinical similarities between chronic fatigue syndrome and depression may be due to a similar distribution of defects in the two disorders.

A comparable study from Belgium (41) studied the clinical correlates of SPECT scans in patients with CFS, major depression and healthy controls. Rather surprisingly, in contrast to the findings of the previous study and in other studies using SPECT, as well as those studies using other techniques, it was reported *"There is neither a global nor a marked regional hypoperfusion in CFS compared with healthy controls,"* a finding which is in marked contrast to the published findings of Mena and Goldstein. Despite this finding, it was observed that *"A lower superfrontal perfusion index is demonstrated in major depression compared with both chronic fatigue syndrome and healthy controls."* But that statement is at variance with the claim that *"Patients with chronic fatigue syndrome and depression had similar numbers of defects per patient."* It is possible that differences in diagnosis of CFS are responsible for the Belgian finding being so different from the findings of others.

A more recent report from Brazil (42) described the use of SPECT to study the relationship between rCBF and separate symptom clusters in major depression. The authors hypothesised that "...*the functional activity in frontal, parietal, anterior cingulate, basal ganglia and limbic regions would be related to specific symptom domains.*" The study involved fifteen patients with major depressive disorder (MDD) and fifteen normal volunteers. It was found that symptom severity correlated with rCBF in different regions, and the authors concluded

> *Our findings confirmed the prediction that separate symptom domains of the MDD syndrome are related to specific rCBF patterns and extend results from prior studies that suggested the involvement of anterior cingulate, frontal, limbic and basal ganglia regions in the pathophysiology of MDD.*

In their PET-based study, Dolan et al (33) reached the similar conclusion that "...symptomatic specificity may be ascribed to regional functional deficits in major depressive illness."

From a wider viewpoint, the findings of Lucey et al (34) imply that if the "regional functional deficits" are sufficiently severe, then they may become manifest as separate psychological/psychiatric disorders.

What this brief review indicates is that irrespective of the technique used to assess cerebral blood flow in depressive illness, the common finding is that rCBF is reduced. Furthermore, some symptoms are relatable to reduced rates of blood flow in specific brain regions.

A rather surprising feature of these studies is the lack of discussion of what factor or factors were responsible for the demonstrated reductions in rCBF, even though only a small number of factors determine capillary blood flow. Of the three major factors, one (capillary diameter) is fixed, while two (blood viscosity, red cell deformability) are variable, although with different time frames.

The published results, which show regions with reduced rates of blood flow, are compatible with the suggestion in 1992 (43) that in the presence of shape-changed, poorly deformable red cells, symptoms could relate to the presence of clusters of smaller than usual capillaries.

In such circumstances, agents which improve red cell deformability could have therapeutic value by increasing the rate of capillary blood flow. Of the various agents which might be useful, most information relates to evening primrose oil, fish oil and pentoxifylline, all of which have been shown to improve red cell deformability when taken in sufficient quantities. Although there are many published reports relating to the use of fish oil in depressive illness, none referred to the effects on red cell deformability, and there was no acknowledgement of the report by Kamada et al (44) which showed that sardine oil increased the fluidity of the red cell membrane lipid bilayer. No reports of the use of evening primrose oil or pentoxifylline in the treatment of depressive illness were located. The reported increase in regional blood flow in the post-depression state, by Bench et al, (37) is the type of change which would be expected if red cell deformability had been improved.

142

Thus it seems that the chance event of Komaroff et al (20) choosing multiple sclerosis and depression as "comparison groups," in a study of CFS, has led to the possibility that all three disorders have similar aetiologies, based primarily on the idiosyncratic presence of smaller than usual capillaries in different regions of the body, and the presence of shape-changed, poorly deformable red cells.

The changes in red cell shape populations are the consequence of any event which alters the internal environment, such as hormonal changes or the immune responses to infections of viruses or bacteria, or to exposure to toxins. Much effort has been expended in trying to identify a specific virus in CFS but it is more likely that it is the responses to the viruses, rather than the virus per se, which are the cause of the problem.

The effects of impaired blood flow seem to be most severe in multiple sclerosis, where the shape-changed red cells may lead to focal ischemic necrosis, followed by plaque formation, with the locality of the lesion determining the nature of the outcome and the severity of disability.

In contrast, both CFS and depression are not associated with tissue damage and have the capacity to re-establish normal tissue function. Although there is no published information about red cell shape in depressive illness, changed shape populations are present in MS and in ME. It will be noted later that changed red cell shape populations occur also in CFIDS, CFS and in fibromyalgia. Therefore it is very likely that depressive illness will be shown to have this feature also.

A consequence of the widespread adoption of the label 'CFS' was the development of a variety of biochemical tests which purported to provide relevant information about the disorder. While the claims made about such tests were of dubious value, there is good evidence that many people had the tests, with obvious financial benefits for their proponents. But in terms of Ramsay's concepts, if the test results were abnormal, then ME would not have been involved.

In a recent article, Myhill et al (59) linked CFS to mitochondrial dysfunction, and reported the development of an "ATP profile" test, in people with CFS selected on the basis of the CDC criteria. Although there was recognition of the need for oxygen and nutrient substrates to sustain normal tissue function, there was no mention of the need for normal rates of blood flow. However, it was noted that "...*blood flow and vascular abnormalities such as orthostatic intolerance (vascular system) ....was one of the clinical abnormalities that define CFS.*"

In a discussion of *"Mitochondrial energy metabolism"* there was no indication that a reduction in the rate of blood flow would have an adverse effect on mitochondrial function, even though a switch to anaerobic respiration in athletes was discussed.

In the website http://www.drmyhill.co.uk Dr. Myhill wrote about "Chronic fatigue syndrome the central cause: mitochondrial failure." In the introduction she stated

> *A very useful analogy is to think of the body as a car. What supplies the energy and the power to make the car work is the engine. Effectively, mitochondria are the engines of our cells – they supply the energy necessary for all cellular processes to take place.*

But the engine will not work if there is no fuel, which draws attention to the need for blood flow to provide the substrates for intracellular processes. However, according to the website of the United Mitochondrial Disease Foundation

> *The conventional teaching in biology and medicine is that mitochondria function only as "energy factories" for the cell. This over-simplification is a mistake which has slowed our progress toward understanding the biology underlying mitochondrial disease.*

The Foundation website stated

> *Mitochondrial diseases are the result of either inherited or spontaneous mutations in mitochondrial DNA or normal DNA which lead to altered functions of the proteins or RNA molecules that normally reside in the mitochondria.*

This genetic interpretation of mitochondrial function is totally different from Dr. Myhill's claim that mitochondria need to be fed, and calls into question the relevance of the nutrient supplements which she claims are necessary. It was proposed that CFS, "...*is the* **symptom** (my emphasis) *caused by mitochondrial failure"*. In the explanation of how every cell in the body can be affected, it was proposed that it was the recycling time for ATP which determines the stamina of an individual. There was no recognition of the need in "oxidative phosphorylation" for a minimum rate of delivery of oxygen, which would relate directly to the rate of capillary blood flow.

This failure to recognise the need for adequate rates of capillary blood flow is evident in the "Treatment package for failing mitochondria," which has four main factors; pacing, feeding the mitochondria, addressing the underlying causes and addressing the secondary damage caused by mitochondrial failure.

In feeding the mitochondria, it was considered necessary to, "...*supply the raw material necessary for the mitochondria to heal themselves and work efficiently."* But this assumes that the delivery system (blood flow) is functional and adequate. Even though impaired blood flow is a potentially limiting factor for mitochondrial function, this was not discussed. The failure to recognise the need for a functional delivery system to "feed" the mitochondria raises questions about the claim that the perfect test is the "ATP profile" test which is considered as a measure of mitochondrial function. In addition to that test, six other tests are added to produce a "Mitochondrial Function Profile." The cost of the tests is £275 which includes a £70 payment for a letter to the patient's GP, and cheques were made payable to Sarah Myhill Limited. The costs involved give rise to the question of whether or not this is the most recent attempt to explain CFS in biochemical terms at great cost to sufferers. Just how mitochondrial dysfunction could relate to remissions is unclear, so the work may be irrelevant for people with ME.

In a discussion of a paper by Dr. Peckerman, it was rather surprising to read of the effects of blood flow in different tissues (the skin, muscles, liver and gut, brain and heart). But all conditions in those tissues were considered to be suitable for treatment of mitochondrial problems, and the treatment involved the use of a package of supplements which "support" mitochondria. The package included, "...D-ribose, CoQ10, acetyl-1-carnitine, NAD, magnesium and B12 injections," so the treatment would not be cheap.

A discussion of "Severe chronic fatigue syndrome" included the statement, "If the heart is in a low output state, then blood supply is poor and therefore the fuel and oxygen necessary to make the engine work are also impaired." Rather surprisingly, this is the only recognition of the fact that a lack of oxygen is considered to have an effect. As SPECT scans have shown reduced rates or regional cerebral blood flow, the crucial question which needs to be addressed is whether or not mitochondria can function normally regardless of the rate of delivery of oxygen. It would seem very likely that mitochondrial dysfunction is the consequence of an inadequate rate of blood flow rather than a primary event.

CFS versus ME: 1997-2007

Continued international interest in CFS and ME/CFS or CFS/ME was manifested by the publication of many papers (it has been stated that more than 5000 papers have been published) dealing with various aspects of the problem. The main points of interest involved immune dysfunction, post-viral or post-infection states and the effects of exercise. The failure to obtain any significant information relating to aetiology or pathogenesis from such a large input into research could be interpreted as indicating that the research was based upon erroneous concepts or that there was a lack of uniformity in the status of the patient panels studied. In other words, apples were not being compared with apples.

In 1997, I published an invited paper titled, "Myalgic encephalomyelitis (ME): a haemorheological disorder manifested as impaired blood flow," (45) and in the text I stated that other chronic disorders with the symptoms of persistent tiredness and easy exhaustibility (MS, AIDS, Occupational Overuse Syndrome, SLE, type 1 and type 2 diabetes, leprosy, post-polio syndrome, Gulf War Syndrome and arachnoiditis) were associated with changed shape populations of red blood cells. Therefore it needs to be emphasised that red cell shape is NOT a diagnostic feature of ME.

> To clarify that statement, Dr. Simpson is saying that ME cannot be diagnosed solely on the basis of shape-changed populations of red blood cells. As stated elsewhere, his view is that once the Ramsay diagnostic criteria have been met (including diagnosis by exclusion), then electron micrographs of immediately fixed red blood samples showing a large proportion of shape-changed cells could serve to *support* a diagnosis of ME.

Changed shape populations of red cells are indicators of a problem of capillary blood flow, which may be temporary in healthy subjects but persistent in those suffering from chronic disorders. What is important is that it may be possible, by the use of appropriate agents, to make the red cells more deformable and to thus increase the rate of blood flow in capillaries and improve tissue function.

Throughout this decade, much time and effort was devoted to the development of "guidelines" for general practitioners, even though there was no agreed upon pathophysiology which would provide an informed basis for management and treatment.

Before examining the various guideline studies, it needs to be stated that a benefit from my extensive travelling to speak to ME groups, was that it resulted in large numbers of blood samples. Almost two thousand two hundred women who were members of ME groups in four countries provided me with blood samples and the analysis of the results have been published. (46).

Because blood samples from the USA came with a variety of labels – CFS, FM, CFS/FM, FM/CFIDS, CFIDS/ME, together with one hundred and six without such designations, six hundred and twenty-three American samples were analysed separately (47). For unexplained reasons, during my later visits there were increasing numbers of people with a diagnosis of fibromyalgia (FM), and the results from six hundred and twenty-three FM blood samples have been published (48). The implications from these findings were published in 2001 in a short paper titled, "On the pathophysiology of ME/CFS" (49).

The Australian Guidelines

The first draft of a document titled, "Chronic fatigue syndrome; clinical practice guidelines; exposure draft," was released by the Royal Australasian College of Physicians (RACP) in December 1997, with a request for comments to be received by February 16, 1998.

The contents of the draft were soon under attack from various sources, and it was not until May 2002 that a larger version comprising sixty-seven pages and five hundred and twenty-eight cited references was published (50). It is of interest that it was stated "'*CFS' is a descriptive term used to define a recognisable pattern of symptoms that cannot be attributed to any alternative condition*" a statement not greatly different from Ramsay's concept of ME, but very different from the inclusive nature of the Fukuda et al criteria of 1994.

An interesting feature was the adoption of quality-of-evidence ratings, which in effect, allowed for a degree of censorship as the decision to cite a reference was, "...*according to the rigour of the research methods used.*" The highest level of research quality, "...*represents consensus opinions of experts, including working group members, based upon clinical experience and limited data.*" But as none of the working group had contributed to the field of blood rheology, it was not surprising that not one of my papers was cited. Rather surprisingly, Professor Campbell Murdoch's studies also failed to be recognised. But of the seventy-odd papers published in the book by Hyde, Goldstein and Levine, only one paper was cited; the paper by Loblay and Swain, titled, "The role of food intolerance in CFS." It could be relevant that Dr. Loblay was the co-convenor of the RACP working party.

However, the paper was important with regard to a statement in a section titled "Pathogenesis," which noted

> *Clinically there are several striking features of chronic fatigue syndrome compared with the paucity of physical signs; the absence of significant immunopathology; the fluctuating course (both short-term and long-term); the occurrence of spontaneous remissions (occasionally full recovery) even after prolonged illness; and the lack of long-term progression in most cases.*

146

This is one of the only two references to remissions made in the book. The other reference was by Dr. Peter Snow. But remissions seem not to relate to CFS, and are never discussed by American investigators. However, as remissions are a feature of ME, does this imply that Loblay and Swain were working with ME people? In addition, the statement challenges the American concept of immune system dysfunction as a major factor in CFS.

Despite the recognition of remissions in the 1992 publication, there is no discussion of remissions in the 2002 Guidelines although in a section dealing with 'Physical activity,' a reference was made to "good days," which could be recognition of remissions. It was stated *"The pathophysiological basis of CFS is unclear"* but of six possibilities discussed, there was no reference to problems of blood flow, which implies the rejection of Ramsay's concepts. But with regard to diagnosis, came this rather surprising statement: *"Diagnosis relies upon the presence of characteristic symptoms and exclusion of alternative medical and psychiatric disorders"* which is similar to Ramsay's criteria for a diagnosis of ME.

In a section titled, "Brain structure/function," it was noted that white- matter abnormalities had been observed by MRI and that SPECT studies had produced conflicting results, but the nature of the conflict was not discussed. When "Psychological/psychiatric factors," were discussed, an interesting comment stated

> *Several lines of evidence suggest that a disturbance of central nervous system function is present in people with CFS. This disturbance is reversible and, as yet is poorly characterised. The pattern of alteration seen in people with CFS in these studies contrasts with that seen in major depression, suggesting different pathophysiological processes in these two syndromes.*

Such a statement probably arises from the idea that SPECT studies had produced conflicting results, but an exploration of the literature would have led to reports which show that SPECT-demonstrated disturbance of central nervous system function, as occurs in depressive illness, closely resembles the SPECT scans seen in CFS. Both in CFS and in depressive illness, the differences in the regions of regional cerebral blood flow appear to relate to the manifestation of different symptoms.

Although it was claimed that *"Muscle strength and recovery are normal,"* several of the quoted studies used "static" exercise, which has been shown to produce results which are different from the effects of "dynamic" exercise. **A major benefit from low intensity exercise is a reduction in blood viscosity, whereas high-intensity exercise changes the shape populations of red cells and increases blood viscosity**. The systemic effects of intense exercise have been demonstrated by Goldstein, who showed that post-exercise SPECT of CFS patients, showed a greater reduction in regional cerebral blood flow than in a pre-exercise scan.

In a later section titled "How should fatigue be evaluated?" seven associated symptoms and signs were listed and included myalgia, loss of concentration, memory impairment and post-exertional malaise. It was stated *"Any of these associated features may be exacerbated by minor physical activity."* But such functional changes are the expected consequences when exercise-induced changes in red cell shape are added to an existing abnormal level.

Under the heading, "Poisoning," it was stated that an illness resembling CFS may develop when the levels of chlorinated hydrocarbons are increased; or following chronic exposure to industrial solvents, insecticides and pesticides; that similar changes may follow silicone breast implants, and that ciguatera poisoning may precipitate a syndrome resembling CFS.

The common feature in all these conditions is that they change the internal environment and would thus stimulate changes in the red cell shape populations. Furthermore, it is very likely that in the case of an individual who manifests symptoms, both the symptoms and their severity will be related to the presence of smaller-than-usual capillaries. This implies that although all those exposed to the toxic agents will have shape-changed red cells, only those with small capillaries will manifest persisting symptoms. But there was no discussion about the significance of the observation that two agents were associated with illnesses which resembled CFS.

In discussing, "What is the natural history of fatigue states?" it was stated *"Outcome has not been found to be associated with sex or life stress events."* But there is considerable evidence that both mental and physical stress can trigger relapses. So it is important to recognise that the stress hormones (catecholamines) were reported to reduce red cell deformability in 1975 (25).

Under the heading, "What is known about the pathophysiology of CFS?" six hypotheses were summarised as follows:

> ...*a unique pattern of infection with a recognised or novel pathogen; altered central nervous system functioning resulting from an abnormal immune response against a common antigen; a neuroendocrine disturbance; a neuropsychiatric disorder with clinical and neurobiological aspects suggesting a link to depressive disorders; a psychologically determined response to infection or other stimuli occurring in 'vulnerable' individuals.*

However, the question of what feature might render an individual vulnerable was not discussed.

Strangely there was no mention of Ramsay's "circulatory impairment" and none of these hypotheses appear to recognise the implications of the SPECT studies in CFS which show reduced regional cerebral blood flow, or the similar studies which used SPECT in depressive illness and in psychiatric disorders.

Is it possible that what is called a "neuroendocrine disturbance" is a manifestation of inadequate rates of oxygen and metabolic substrates to sustain normal function in nerve tissue and in endocrine glands? Is it logical to expect any tissue to function normally when impaired capillary blood flow results in an inadequate rate of delivery of substrates?

None of the six hypotheses referred to or addressed the significance of the several reports relating to epidemic outbreaks that relapses were triggered by physical activity, cold weather or the onset of menstruation. The common feature is that all three factors are associated with reduced rates of blood flow.

In a discussion "What is fatigue?" it was concluded that fatigue "...*is intrinsically a brain-mediated sensation*" which implies that the authors were unaware of the

RAMSAY'S DISEASE - ME

physiological concepts of muscle fatigue, as a consequence of inadequate rates of oxygen delivery. The possible role of an inadequate rate of blood flow in fatigue may have been highlighted in a box in which eleven patient-described problems were interpreted. Although multiple sclerosis (which has been shown to have abnormal blood rheology) was only one of the possible interpretations, in no interpretation was an insufficient rate of blood flow considered as a possible causal factor.

The following section, "How should fatigue be evaluated?" listed seven associated symptoms and signs which included myalgia, loss of concentration, memory impairment and post-exertional malaise. It was stated also *"Any of these associated features may be exacerbated by minor physical activity."* But such changes are the expected consequences when activity-induced changes in the shape populations of red cells are added to an existing abnormal red cell shape population, as was reported in 1993 (51).

The section headed "Alternative causes of chronic fatigue" included reference to sixteen different classes of illness with twenty-four specific factors, several of which had been shown to have changed red-cell-shape populations and altered blood rheology. Thus it would seem that in rejecting the possibility that inadequate rates of delivery of oxygen and nutrient substrates may lead to tissue dysfunction, the authors may have made it impossible to understand the nature of fatigue states.

In "What psychological evaluation is required?" it was stated, *"A formal diagnosis of CFS should not be made without an appropriate psychological evaluation of the patient"* and that referral could be useful. An interesting section posed the question, "Should the context of the illness be assessed?" It was suggested that the effects of the illness on the social circumstances and on inter-personal relationships should be considered. An evaluation of such factors may enable doctors to act as advocates for their patient.

The answer to the question "What laboratory tests are appropriate?" was that no specific diagnostic test has emerged. In addition it was stated

> *Many other laboratory procedures have been proposed as 'diagnostic tests' by non-medical or alternative practitioners, but have not been subjected to rigorous evaluation. Such 'tests' (e.g. field blood testing for red cell morphology or 'Candida' identification; stool tests for environmental sensitivity testing) have no basis in evidence and are not recommended.*

It is not clear what was meant by "field blood testing for red cell morphology," as this could relate to either, "live-cell analysis" or to "red-cell-shape analysis."

During "live-cell analysis" patients are able to watch their red cells change shape on a video screen, and the changes are endowed with various diagnostic features. But the changes in cell shape are simply the responses of unfixed cells to changes in the cell environment, under the cover glass, and such changes have no diagnostic or physiological significance.

On the other hand, the red-cell-shape analysis of immediately fixed red cells shows changes in the shape populations of red cells, indicating that capillary blood flow will be impaired. The results are NOT diagnostic, as changed red cell shape populations have been reported in several chronic disorders such as muscular dystrophy (1976), Huntington's Disease (1977) and spinocerebellar degeneration (1983).

Maybe the failure to recognise these early studies is the reason for the rejection of my work, but the demonstration of the existence of shape-changed red cells provides the basis for treatment aimed at improving capillary blood flow.

"Managing patients with CFS," was considered under a variety of headings and it was noted that Cognitive Behavioural Therapy and Graded Exercise Therapy, "...*may be effective for <u>some</u> people with CFS*" (my underlining). However depending upon the patient's "functional capacity," physical and intellectual activities should be 'paced'. For the relief of symptoms "*Antidepressant drugs may be helpful.*" It should be noted that there is no clear basis for the management suggestions, although a 'pacing' lifestyle would be helpful.

In "Principles of management" it was suggested that a management plan be developed through active discussion with the patient.

> *The goal of treatment should be improvement towards and maintenance of maximal achievable functional capacity. While it is very unlikely that any single treatment will provide a 'cure,' current treatment approaches can result in significant reductions in disability over time.*

In general, the uncertainty about the fundamental nature of the disorder is reflected in recommendations to switch from one form of treatment to another, and the use of a variety of drugs to control key symptoms is recommended. It was noted that the patient/doctor relationship would have a significant impact on outcome.

What seems to be important is that there is nothing in the management plan which may be related to the cause of the problem, and this may become complicated by the development of new symptoms.

Because of the apparent lack of knowledge of the aetiopathology of CFS, it is not surprising that in the section, "Pharmacological treatments for CFS," it was stated that "...*no agent has consistently shown long-term efficacy, etc.*" A discussion of "The role of rehabilitation, behavioural and cognitive treatment approaches" concluded

> *On balance, current evidence suggests that rehabilitative, behavioural and cognitive approaches should be an integral component of managing people with CFS......Doctors should ensure that patients are informed of the dangers of prolonged rest and the psychological risks of social isolation.*

Unfortunately, it seems not to be important when patients tell doctors that CBT and GET worsen their symptoms, although to some extent this situation is reflected in the section titled, "Applying management principles." Three models of the disease are proposed: a cognitive behaviour therapy model; a disease education model; a rehabilitation model. But in proposing a 'disease education model' this implies the existence of information about the nature of the disorder. And if such information was available, how would it relate to the other two models?

> As noted elsewhere, the term 'rehabilitation' is appropriate only in relation to an illness or injury from which recovery has already taken place. A programme of rehabilitation undertaken while the disease process is still on-going or the damage from the injury is not healed will delay or even prevent recovery. Patient-controlled pacing allows people who have ME to conduct themselves in a way that can facilitate recovery, while forced exercise regimes are particularly dangerous for people with ME, exacerbating and prolonging disability. The 'refusals and drop-outs' mentioned below, if investigated, as they should have been, are likely to be of people who realised that the proposed programmes of 'rehabilitation' were at best premature and at worst, putting them at risk of protracted and severe worsening of their symptoms.

The discussion of "Limitations of the evidence" included the statement, "Although most have shown short-term or longer-term benefit (or both) improvement has not been observed in all patients in all studies, and, when observed, may be modest." Such observations could be expected if there was a lack of homogeneity in the participants, and it would be influenced by **the absence of the severely unwell** who were unfit to attend a clinic. In addition there were **varying levels of refusals and drop outs**. Tacit recognition of the lack of homogeneous study panels has been manifested as proposals to sub-classify CFS patients, although no such scheme has been adopted generally.

A table headed "Treatments for chronic fatigue syndrome for which scientific evidence is lacking," included fourteen vitamin and mineral supplements and fourteen physical therapies. Of the vitamin supplements, it should be noted that vitamin B12 (as hydroxocobalamin) has been found to be effective, whereas cyanocobalamin, which is used widely in the USA, is generally ineffective. In people with the increased cup forms of acute ME, injections of hydroxocobalamin at ten to fourteen day intervals resulted in a reduction in the numbers of cup forms and less severe symptoms. But for unknown reasons, only 50% of cases respond to the vitamin. It is of interest that in the UK, injections of hydroxocobalamin are a common treatment for persistent tiredness.

Given that the pathophysiology of CFS in adults is not understood, it is rather surprising that several pages should be devoted to "CFS in children and adolescents" where it was noted that in general, the situation in adolescents was highly consistent with the adult situation.

The report concluded with a discussion of "Social and legal issues" as they relate to Australians.

This document is the outcome of a great deal of work by a committee which comprised five immunologists, two general practitioners, a rheumatologist, a neurologist, an occupational medicine physician, a paediatrician and a consultant physician. It could be expected that there would be great variability in their experience with CFS patients.

According to the Preface, the guidelines were aimed at all healthcare professionals "*...involved in managing people with fatigue states,*" and "*...are intended to provide a general guide to best practices.*" It is arguable that this intention has been realised, given the lack of knowledge of the cause or causes, and therefore of how best they might be treated.

The contents of the guidelines document may be summarised as follows:

1. In the general community there is a segment which fits the diagnostic criteria for CFS, although it was not explained why only some individuals develop CFS after various viral infections while the majority have only a brief illness.
2. Possibly, because the diagnostic criteria may include different clinical entities, there is no clear explanation of the cause (or causes) or how their mode of action leads to the development of fatigue.
3. Because of the lack of acceptable evidence of an 'organic' or physical cause of CFS, sufferers from this condition are frequently referred to psychologists/psychiatrists for diagnosis and treatment.
4. It is noted that psychological/psychiatric based treatments are controversial and are not effective, generally.
5. There is no recognition of the physiological concept of muscle fatigue as the result of an inadequate rate of oxygen delivery, and the possibility that impaired capillary blood flow is involved (as shown by SPECT scans), is not considered.
6. It is unclear how the consequences of this costly exercise will be evaluated and how the relevance (or otherwise) will be assessed.

The Chief Medical Officer's Working Group

About a year after the release of the first draft of the Australian Guidelines, on July 16, 1998, The Chief Medical Officer of Great Britain announced the formation of a Working Group on CFS/ME, and the membership and the brief was announced on November 4. The brief of the Working Group was stated as follows:

To review management and practice in the field of CFS/ME with the aim of providing best practice guidance for professionals, patients and carers to improve the quality of care and treatment for people with CFS/ME, in particular to:

- *develop good clinical practice guidance on the healthcare management of CFS/ME for NHS professionals, using best available evidence;*
- *make recommendations for further research into the care and treatment of people with CFS/ME;*
- *identify areas which might require further work and make recommendations to the CMO.*

The very restrictive nature of the brief should be noted, with the noteworthy feature that there was no recommendation to attempt to determine the cause of and the pathogenesis of the problem. It seems reasonable to ask how the Working Group could rationally identify what is best treatment and care of a disease which has no background.

The "Key Group" comprised fifteen individuals, eight of whom were lay people involved in ME groups or as carers, and of the seven physicians, three were psychologists.

The report stated, "The Key Group was responsible for surveying the evidence, developing the main report and agreeing the final recommendations to the CMO." Prior to this it had been stated that, "...a systematic search of the international evidence had been commissioned." In marked contrast to the five hundred and twenty-eight citations in the Australian Guidelines, only sixty-five items were included in the bibliography, but this probably reflects the limited number of publications in the field of **management and treatment. At least twelve papers related to psychology and seven of these came from one group.** Of the material relating to ME which was known to have been published in Australia and New Zealand, only one paper by Lloyd et al was listed.

Fifteen individuals were named as "Key Group observers" and eight individuals as "Childrens' Group observers" with thirty-six members of a Reference Group. An "Editorial team" of five was chaired by Professor A. Hutchinson and included two freelance medical writers.

The chapter, "Evidence from patients," commenced "During the Working Group process, the strongest message received was that patient's voices were not being listened to and understood." From the patients' viewpoint, what was needed was recognition of the presence of a health problem; a diagnosis which led to acceptance and the eventual acknowledgement of the illness. Despite this need, the restrictive brief of the Working Group seems designed to produce a conclusion of this type: "You have an illness which we do not understand, but we recommend the following treatments." Patient groups considered the greatest need was for more healthcare professionals who understood and accepted CFS/ME, and who were willing to listen to and to support patients. Attention was drawn to the existence of the severely unwell who experienced the adverse effects of isolation and who faced many physical barriers in accessing care. The report noted that, "Clinicians who were interested and experienced in CFS/ME were few in number and patchy in location."

The failure of conventional medical care led patients to move to complementary medicine, where the major benefit was that such practitioners listened! In addition, some treatments helped to alleviate symptoms, which led to the statement, "*If we cannot be cured, at least we can be comfortable.*" A patient view was that as Alzheimer's disease was not known as "Chronic forgetfulness syndrome" this could explain why CFS is unpopular and why ME is the patient-preferred term. The report stated

> *Having a loved one affected by CFS/ME has a profound effect on every part of life. Many carers reported that their world felt that it had been 'turned upside down' and they had feelings of despair.*

Later it was noted

> *...some reported supportive GPs who admitted their limited knowledge and 'feeling out of their depth' with the illness, and treated the family with respect. Carers respect honesty and prefer not to be given an over-optimistic prognosis.*

In addressing the "Nature and impact of CFS/ME" it was stated, "Although the disorder is clinically recognisable, CFS/ME assumes many different clinical forms and is highly variable in severity and duration, but lacks specific disease markers." This statement overlooks the fact that prior to the introduction of CFS in 1988 ME was being diagnosed in several countries on the basis of Ramsay's criteria, which required the exclusion of any other possible diagnosis.

While it is true that, "specific disease markers," are lacking, it is relevant that the reports of poor blood filterability, changed red cell morphology and the results from studies using SPECT scans, all draw attention to the probability that capillary blood flow will be impaired. To ignore such information is tantamount to proposing that normal tissue function can persist in the face of subnormal blood flow.

While it might be appropriate to discuss CFS without mentioning remissions, it would be wrong not to mention such changes in ME. One is left to wonder about the possible consequences of the term CFS/ME, and how the discussion would be different if ME/CFS was being discussed.

In a discussion of the term, "encephalomyelitis," no mention was made of the historical background to the term, i.e. that Acheson had noted: *In our present state of ignorance 'encephalomyelitis' seems preferable to 'encephalopathy' because it conveys the suggestion that the disease is infective in origin, which is most certainly the case.*

The Working Group recognised the unsatisfactory nature of the current terminology, which raises the possibility that my proposal to identify ME as Ramsay's Disease (ME) could be timely.

A discussion titled, "Aetiology, pathogenesis and disease associations," noted that it "…reinforces the view that CFS/ME is a heterogeneous condition…….either in its causative factors or in its clinical nature."

In keeping with the idea of a heterogeneous condition it was stated also that

The occurrence of CFS/ME could involve any of seven factors – none of which are mutually exclusive:

1. CFS/ME is an umbrella term for several different illnesses.
2. One (or more) 'core' disorder(s) exist.
3. Several different causative factors trigger a common disease process.
4. The aetiology and/or pathophysiology are multifactorial.
5. Certain factors are necessary but not sufficient to cause CFS/ME.
6. Certain factors can influence individual manifestations or duration.
7. Some features are downstream (secondary) consequences of the primary disease process.

While it is quite likely that several of these statements are relevant, the outcome of this proposal is that it is no different from the conclusion reached in the Australian Guidelines, i.e. *"The pathophysiological basis of CFS is unclear."* The fundamental point which arises from the idea is that, if these seven possibilities represent the 'best knowledge' of the cause of CFS/ME, then the concept does not provide a good basis for managing the disorder.

But imagine the implications if "the trigger of a common disease process" was the effects of change in the internal environment which stimulated changes in the shape populations of red blood cells – as has been reported. And it is noteworthy that although changed red cell shape populations have been reported in muscular dystrophy, Huntington's Disease and spinocerebellar degeneration, there is no clinical recognition of the possible significance of such changes. The point is that in CFS/ME, such changes would

"...influence individual manifestations," in proportion to the frequency and distribution of clusters of small capillaries.

Therefore, while a subject lacking small capillaries would respond to a viral infection with only minor changes, individuals with clusters of small capillaries in different regions of the body will become dysfunctional. The distribution of the resulting symptoms will be determined by the anatomical location of small capillaries, and the severity of the symptoms and the level of dysfunction will relate to the degree to which the flow rate in capillaries is reduced.

At this time it is not known what factor (or factors) determine the duration of the illness, but the occurrence of remissions indicate that the factor (or factors) have the capacity to switch off and on. Although relevant information was published in 1992 and 1997, it is outside the brief of the Working Group.

Five "Predisposing factors" listed were "gender, familial, personality, other disorders, previous mood disorders." There is no doubt that in general, women are more frequently affected by CFS/ME, so it is of interest that outbreaks in Dalston, England, Adelaide, Australia and in Tapanui, New Zealand, reported sex ratios of 1:1. The implications of the different sex ratio remain unexplained. Nor is there any explanation for the dominance of females suffering from CFS/ME, although the suggestion by Spurgin in 1995 that because women have smaller muscles than men, then maybe they also have smaller capillaries could be relevant. However, this reasonable suggestion has not been investigated.

As there is evidence that some personality factors relate to stress, the fact that the stress hormones influence red cell shape could make personality changes a predisposing factor. In the "other disorders" category, irritable bowel syndrome and fibromyalgia are noted. It is relevant that blood samples from more than three hundred people with fibromyalgia had increased flat cells similar in numbers to people with ME. However, an analysis of the symptoms, arranged in decreasing order of severity, showed that whereas the majority of ME people listed tiredness as their first symptom, pain was the first symptom of people with fibromyalgia. As changed red cell shape populations have been found in other chronic disorders, this emphasises the fact that red cell shape analysis is not a diagnostic test for ME. Instead, the results from the test draw attention to the role of impaired blood flow in the pathophysiology of the associated disorder. The common feature between CFS/ME and mood disorders is that in both conditions there is evidence of reduced regional cerebral blood flow as shown by SPECT scans. Perhaps the most enlightening of such studies was the demonstration that in a region in which blood flow was reduced in depression, blood flow was normal after the resolution of the depression.

Five "triggers" were identified, namely, infections, immunisations, life events, physical injuries and environmental toxins. Again, the factor in common is that all the triggers alter the internal environment leading to changes in the shape populations of red blood cells. Rather surprisingly it was stated, *"The evidence that life events can trigger CFS/ME is weak,"* as it is not uncommon to meet ME people whose ME was the consequence of a life event such as the sudden death of a loved one, or a very stressful divorce. In 1975 it was reported that catecholamines (the stress hormones) reduced the deformability of red blood cells. As Acheson's 1959 paper is listed in the bibliography, it could have been expected that the agents which he recorded as common causes of relapses (cold weather, untimely over-activity, the onset of menstruation) would have been considered as "triggers." While cold weather increases blood viscosity, the other causes of relapses are associated with changes in the shape populations of red cells. Because those changes will be additive to any pre-existing change it can be anticipated that they will be accompanied by a worsening of symptoms, particularly in the premenstrual week.

In the section titled, "Maintaining factors," seven topics are listed: sleep disturbance, mood disorders, inactivity, over-activity, inter-current stressors, iatrogenic illness, and illness beliefs. Although each topic is discussed there is no indication of a common factor which might explain how they "maintain" CFS/ME. But apart from the claimed role of "illness beliefs", the remaining six factors either result from or are causes of changed red cell shape populations. Brain dysfunction follows inadequate rates of delivery of oxygen, so mood problems and sleep disturbance can be expected. SPECT scans in CFS/ME and in depressive illness reveal reduced rates of regional cerebral blood flow, but in different regions. Inactivity is associated with an increase in blood viscosity, which is reduced by regular, low-intensity activity such as walking. On the other hand, energetic activity changes the shape populations of red cells, in both healthy and unwell individuals. As the overall effects of over-activity will be related to the level of intensity and the time involved, the degree of symptom-worsening will be related to the baseline values of red cell shape populations as they will be added to the effects of activity. Stressful situations, both emotional and physical and other health events, probably worsen symptoms through their effects on red cell shape populations and therefore on the rate of capillary blood flow.

It was noted that the psychological concept of "illness beliefs," remains, "...*a contentious issue.*" To a large extent, because a patient firmly believes his/her illness to have a physical cause, the idea that this belief will be an obstacle to treatment may simply reflect the lack of an accepted pathophysiology.

Possible "Disease mechanisms" are discussed under the following headings: biomedical model, bio-psychosocial model, immune, hypothalamic-pituitary-adrenal axis, central nervous system, peripheral and autonomic nervous system. **My findings leave me in no doubt that the only relevant disease mechanism is the biomedical model as this fits well with Simpson's Axiom, "Persistently impaired capillary blood flow is totally incompatible with normal tissue function."**

The report stated

> In this over-arching conceptual framework, CFS/ME is seen as a condition like many other medical conditions where illness results from a specific pathologic defect in physiological functioning, mediated at organ, tissue, cellular and/or molecular level, by as yet undetermined mechanisms. It is not incompatible with the following (i.e. bio-psychosocial model) but implies that a primary disease entity exists and that bio-psychosocial aspects are consequential.

In view of the demonstrated problems of blood flow, this statement stimulates the question: is normal 'physiological functioning' at any level possible when the rate of blood flow is greatly reduced? For example, consider the implications if the "*...as yet undefined mechanism*" was impaired capillary blood flow? **The major obstacle to this concept is that the science involved (haemorheology/blood rheology) is not taught at medical schools.** But blood with increased viscosity, containing shape-changed, poorly deformable red cells, would affect "*...physiological functioning, mediated at organ, tissue, cellular and/or molecular levels.*" Because the nature of the microcirculation will be idiosyncratic, regions supplied by small capillaries may range from near zero to body-wide, and **for that reason there is no need to complicate the situation by the introduction of psychological concepts**. By altering the internal environment, immunological abnormalities will contribute to the blood flow problems in the microcirculation. Because it is known that nerve cells, muscle cells and endocrine glands are particularly sensitive to deprivation of their metabolic needs (particularly oxygen and nutrient substrates) such tissues would be the first to be affected by altered blood rheology. For this reason it would not be surprising if there was disruption of the hypothalamic-pituitary-adrenal axis. However, the authors of the report appear not to recognise the fundamental importance of normal blood flow, as the report states "*One suggested primary change in the central nervous system of patients with CFS/ME is abnormal blood flow, particularly involving the brainstem. However, many of these findings are inconsistent.*" This is an obvious reference to the SPET study of Dr. D.C. Costa, which was reported first at the annual general meeting of the British Nuclear Medicine Society on March 30, 1994. Although he reported that the brainstem blood flow in ME/CFS people was lower than in those with depression, the rate of blood flow in both disorders was significantly lower than in healthy subjects. However, what the Working Group failed to note was that Dr. Costa also reported "*...a generalised reduction in brain perfusion.*" As the report downplays the implications of such studies, making no reference to the earlier work of Mena, Goldstein and Hyde in this field, this raises the question of why the topic was raised in the first place.

As both ME and CFS patients have altered red cell shape populations and suffer from cognitive problems, the question arises, is there a parallel with Huntington's Disease? In 1977 it was reported (52) that the blood of Huntington's Disease patients contained high numbers of stomatocytes (cup forms) which occur also in acute ME. In 1985, without reference to the findings of the 1977 study, Tanahashi et al (53) reported that Huntington's Disease patients had reduced cerebral blood flow which correlated with the results from cognitive testing.

The section titled, "Spectrum of illness," had some interesting observations under the headings "subgroups, symptom profiles, severity." In "subgroups" it was stated

> *The issue of subgroups or distinct entities within CFS/ME was the subject of much debate by the Working Group. We are conscious that some sectors strongly hold the view that the term ME defines a subgroup within CFS, or even a distinct condition. The Working Group accepts that some patients' presentation and symptoms align more closely to the original clinical description of ME than to the current definition of CFS by the Centres for Disease Control and Prevention. However, there is currently no clear scientific evidence to allow formal*

157

differentiation of ME from CFS on the basis of pathophysiology or response to treatment. Therefore, for the purposes of this report, we regard CFS/ME as a single, albeit diverse, clinical entity.

Again, the Working Group disregards the fact that in several countries ME was a diagnosable condition prior to the confusion which followed the introduction of CFS. The 1988 guidelines were widened in 1994, and the apparent determination of the Americans to confuse the issue was marked in early 2007 when a group decided to change CFS to ME.

It is unclear just what message the following statement was intended to convey: "We hold the view that every patient's experience is unique and his or her illness must be treated flexibly in its own right, from a range of options that are generally applicable to the disorder but individually adapted. This approach is similar to that for many other conditions." Possibly, this is related to the decision that ME and CFS are the same condition, even though CFS is recognised as being a heterogeneous disorder, but the relevance of the statement remains unclear.

The section "Symptom profiles" began, "Patients with CFS/ME experience an individual array of symptoms from the range seen in the illness. Some, such as physical and/or cognitive fatigue are seen in almost all patients, though their extent may vary. Others are very common, such as pain, disturbed sleep and gastrointestinal disturbance."

But in the lists of symptoms which came with more than thirteen thousand blood samples, the term 'fatigue' was used rarely, with tiredness being the most common descriptor. This is in accord with the experience of Sir John Ellis who in 1984 noted that fatigue and malaise were textbook terms which were seldom used by patients.

However, a discussion of symptoms without any concept of causation was unsatisfactory, although it was noted that menstrual exacerbation of symptoms had been reported. To a major degree, the lack of knowledge about their symptoms and their variability were causes of alarm and frustration, which impacted also on family and carers. It was stated "*Anxiety or depression, anger and withdrawal from social interaction are relatively common consequences in response to the impact of any chronic illness on personal and social functioning. These understandable reactions add to distress, and in some cases become part of, or even dominate, the clinical picture of CFS/ME.*" In such circumstances it is easy to imagine the benefits of meeting with a supportive GP, who, after listening to the patient's story, says, "Look, I do not fully understand the nature of your problem, so let you and I work on it."

The same problems concerning symptoms were to a considerable extent manifested in the section titled "Severity," as any assessment of severity would be personal. Although a four-category level of severity was quoted, the classification related to functional ability, rather than symptom severity per se. It was noted

Such patients may suffer most impact through the discrepancy between what they were able to achieve previously and what they can do now. Even less prolonged illness, whatever the severity, can have substantial personal and social impact, mainly intrusions on the individual, relationships, work and finances. Self-confidence and self-esteem are severely eroded in many cases.

Although the expression of multiple symptoms is the norm, it is not uncommon to find a patient whose quality of life is eroded by the persistence and severity of a single symptom.

A subsection "People with severe disease" probably reflected the contributions from groups such as 25%ME and CHROME. It was stated *"Current provision of services falls well below what is needed for the vast majority of severely and very severely affected patients."* It was recognised that many would not be able, physically, to take advantage of available services, and that *"Severe illness that continues over many years with no sense of improvement has a profound cumulative personal and social impact"* and that *"Those who are most severely affected need acknowledgement, encouragement, and support to remain optimistic."*

To a large extent, the section "Socioeconomic impact" was stating the obvious, i.e. that not being able to work has serious social consequences which will be worsened to the degree of monetary obligations such as the need to service a mortgage. Financial obligations not infrequently stimulate a premature return to work with a resulting exacerbation of symptoms.

In addition "Patients can encounter arbitrary and poorly informed decision-making on other issues such as home help and mobility badge schemes, as well as sheer resource limitations."

> The irony, for an ME sufferer applying for a mobility badge, at least in the UK, is that eligibility depends on your being 'permanently disabled'. A person suffering from ME who is able to minimise the risk of overexertion in the early stages is less likely to become 'permanently disabled'. But there is no understanding that having a mobility badge might help **prevent** disability becoming 'permanent'.

The effects of such failure to gain access to social support programs "...can be compounded if doctors fail to provide clear guidance about diagnosis and need."

Perhaps the most significant feature of this section on the "Nature and impact of CFS/ME," was the decision to reject ME as a clinical entity. Even if ME represented only 5% of CFS/ME, the separation from the heterogeneous concept of CFS would have provided a more definable target for investigations. However, the impact of ME is unlikely to be greatly different from that defined for CFS/ME.

The first ten pages of the chapter on 'Management of CFS/ME' are devoted mainly to recognition and diagnosis as a part of management. A primary problem for the Working Group was the divergence of opinion concerning the nature of CFS/ME, and those differing views would influence management. It was noted specifically that the aim was not to produce a consensus but to delineate the differences where they existed.

In "Recognition, acknowledgement and acceptance" it was stated that the lack of these factors could have an adverse effect on both patients and carers. Healthcare professionals were encouraged to adopt an understanding attitude by listening to the patient and that by recognising and accepting the patient's experience, they could develop a positive relationship. An early agreement concerning a name for the illness was deemed to be important.

The "Approach to management" was hindered by the lack of an accepted pathophysiology, and it was stated "No management approach to CFS/ME has been found to be universally beneficial, etc." While "Most people with CFS/ME can expect some degree of improvement with time and treatment," the nature and objective of the treatment was not discussed. But it is debatable that "A multi-disciplinary assessment is key to the provision of a supportive package of health care and social care provision," as this implies the assessment will provide useful relevant information.

In "Diagnosis and evaluation" the proposed unitary nature of CFS/ME is reflected in the statement "*CFS/ME should be treated in the same way as any other chronic illness of unknown aetiology.*" But, given the heterogeneous nature of CFS, is this suggestion reasonable?

The "Diagnostic process" recognised the importance for patients and carers to have an early diagnosis and a name for the illness. Rather strangely, it was recommended that "*A positive diagnosis of CFS/ME is needed rather than one of exclusion*" as this seems to reflect upon Ramsay's use of exclusion of other diagnoses in his ME criteria. In addition, in the absence of a recognised marker for CFS/ME, it has been stated that the diagnosis "*...is based on recognition of a typical symptom pattern together with exclusion of alternative conditions.*" However, given the wide range of symptoms and their variability in expression, defining a "typical symptom pattern" would not be a simple procedure. To some extent this is reflected in the suggestion that "*CFS/ME should be considered at an early stage as part of the differential diagnosis where individuals of **any age** (my emphasis) present with symptoms of excessive tiredness or fatigue*" but this fails to recognise that a part of the aging process are changes in blood rheology. Persisting with the idea that "*...symptoms start to form a recognisable pattern ... some investigations may be undertaken, which is considered appropriate when other diagnoses have been excluded.*"

Possibly because of the limitations of the Working Group's brief, it was noted that investigations "...that may improve our understanding of aetiology and pathogenesis, and better treatment; (are) restricted, as, ...such clinical research, with appropriate consent is important, but it must be explicitly distinguished from normal clinical care." It seems peculiar that in a section headed, "Diagnostic process," the search for the cause of the problem seems not to be a primary objective.

This apparent confusion continues in the following section, "Diagnostic criteria" which commences "Current diagnostic criteria are useful only for research purposes, and no clinically recognised set of diagnostic criteria exists."

The concept of exclusion is raised again in the statement "A diagnosis of CFS/ME (but without a set of diagnostic criteria – my comment) as with other chronic illnesses of uncertain aetiology relies on the presence of a set of characteristic symptoms, together with the exclusion of alternative diagnoses."

While it was noted that in the early stages of the illness there is an, "*...intolerance to both physical and mental exertion,*" there was no discussion of the nature of the intolerance. It was noted that "persistent fatigue" (not defined) needed to be differentiated from "acute fatigue," but without any comment on the difference.

Perhaps the most significant feature of this section was the final sentence: "Another distinguishing feature of the illness, (CFS/ME) in comparison with other 'fatigue states' is its **prolonged relapsing and remitting course** (my emphasis) over months or years." This draws attention to the nearly nonsensical approaches to the discussion of the "Diagnostic process" and "Diagnostic criteria" neither of which mention remissions, despite the obvious implications of such changes, with particular regard to any proposed pathophysiology. While Ramsay's criteria for ME recognise the occurrence of remissions, such events are not a recognised part of CFS, and to a considerable extent this emphasises the problem created by choosing to use the term CFS/ME.

The lack of clarity of thought persists into the section, "Characteristic features," which noted the following symptoms; "…overwhelming fatigue, related effects on both physical and cognitive functioning, and malaise, typically exacerbated by a wide range of other symptoms." Even though it has been noted that it is unusual for patients to use the term fatigue, it was stated "The fatigue is commonly described as like no other in type and severity, and is evidently very different from everyday tiredness." But the first of a list of seven characteristic or common symptoms was, "Persistent/excessive tiredness or fatigue."

A major problem in the section, "Onset and course," is the lack of recognition of the role of infections and other triggers in changing the flow properties of blood. It was recognised that there was a role for other triggers, which is apparent in the statement "*The importance of such factors in the population burden of CFS/ME is unclear.*" There is no apparent recognition that "triggers" exert their influence by changing the internal environment, which will affect the shape and deformability of red blood cells.

In discussing, "Predictors of chronicity," the major obstacle was the lack of utilisable information, leading to some speculation. Of particular interest is the listing of three important factors as, "*Other factors that appear to be associated with poor prognosis.*" The first of these, "*…the coexistence of psychiatric and other chronic illnesses with CFS/ME*" seems to imply that the diagnosis has been made without excluding alternative diagnoses.

The second factor "*…a long duration of symptoms of CFS/ME,*" would seem to be self-evident. But the third factor, "*…older age,*" is the probable manifestation of the fact that the aging process is associated with increased blood viscosity (54) and the existence of shape-changed, poorly deformable red cells to which would be added the red cell shape changes of CFS/ME. It has been reported that blood samples from people aged between 60 and 96 years have high levels of flat cells, (55) with values similar to those found in chronic ME.

In "Clinical evaluation" it was noted that the purpose of the exercise was "… to increase the probability of a correct diagnosis of CFS/ME; to rule out other conditions; to confirm the diagnosis; to identify any clinical sub-grouping relevant to the patient; and to identify and characterise clinically significant consequences." While these are obviously desirable objectives, there is no comment relating to remissions, so it needs to be asked, "What other disorders present with a, '…prolonged relapsing and remitting course over months or years"?

The section "Information and support" provides some common sense observations about the effects of uncertainty on patients, carers and physicians. Although the information needs of patients may be different from those of carers and family members, in general all need to know what options exist; what progress can be expected and what is the long term prognosis? It was stated *"Information on the nature of the condition and self-management seems to facilitate adjustments to the illness and a better outcome. Such education is also particularly important for anticipating and managing fluctuations or more substantial remissions or relapses."* This is only the second mention of remissions in forty-one pages and it raises several questions, particularly in the context of a section "Information and support," as on the same page is a box headed, "Patient's questions that clinicians can answer," containing the following statements:

- Initially, whether they are ill and what their illness is.
- Is it their fault? Are they getting old, going mad, developing Alzheimer's disease, etc.
- Will it get worse? If they improve will they relapse?
- Which treatments are worth trying?
- How will others react?
- To whom can they safely talk about how they feel?
- What will the impact of their illness be on them, their work, or their friends and family relationships?
- How will they cope financially? Can they work?

It is unacceptable to claim that clinicians should be able to answer such questions as they pose such a variety of imponderables. Take the first question for example. How does a clinician explain to a patient that they have a disorder of which the cause and nature is unknown, but there may be a variety of symptoms which show variable levels of severity? In addition there may be periods of remission which may last for hours, days, weeks or months and there is no recognised and acceptable treatment. The honest answer to most of the questions would be, "I do not know."

In discussing, "Self-management," it was stated that the successful management of long-term illness involves the taking of the patient as a partner in care. This would involve education, so that the patient became an expert in his or her condition. However, it is unclear how psychologists would regard such 'illness beliefs.' In my experience, ME people avidly examine all available information about their illness, within the constraints of their illness-impaired mental capabilities. But in the absence of any understanding of the cause of the problem and the variable time frame of remissions and relapses, it may be very difficult to apply self-management strategies.

"Equipment and practical assistance," draws attention, to how those suffering from chronic illnesses, may be helped by *"…sympathetic provision of appropriate practical assistance."* But, given the fluctuating levels of capability, establishing the nature of such assistance will not be a simple matter.

A consideration of "Support to family carers" included a box, headed "Carer's questions that clinicians can answer" which included the following questions:

- Will they need to leave their jobs?

- How long will the illness last, and how disabled will their loved one be, during this time?
- What can the carer do and what should they not do?
- Will their doctors believe them?
- Where can they get advice about benefits?

While there is no doubt that the clinician would be able to answer the last question, it is very unlikely that a clinician could provide useful answers to the remaining questions. The authors of the report are being most unfair to clinicians in implying that they can predict the course of the illness.

The discussion of "Ongoing care" seemed not to recognise the full implications, for a patient suffering from a relapsing/remitting disorder. An assessment of available evidence concerning the effectiveness of treatments noted a paucity of good quality evidence.

A section headed "People who are severely affected" was probably stimulated by the contributions from groups such as 25%ME and CHROME, as it stated *"Not enough is known about severe forms of the condition CFS/ME that are reported to affect 25% of patients."* Although the Working Group was aware *"…that provision for health care for these severely affected patients is often seriously inadequate……we found insufficient evidence available to guide specific management of those people who are severely affected."* Possibly due to the knowledgeable contribution by the 25%ME representatives, the problems of the severely ill were given more than usual attention.

On reflecting on the absence of knowledge relating to causation, it was stated "It seems best, on present evidence, to recognise the need to adapt therapies to the functional level of the patient, and to adjust them further in response to feedback from the patient during therapy." In other words, patients did have an opinion on how they were affected by any therapy. In order to utilise the information obtained during treatment of other chronic disorders, it was stated "Healthcare and social service professionals are responsible for finding ways of supporting and guiding patients and their carers for the duration of illness, ensuring access to available support, keeping in contact, constantly re-evaluating the options, maintaining morale, enabling respite and minimising the consequences of prolonged disease." There would be little complaint if such objectives involved all CFS/ME patients, but there is significant information which shows that such good intentions have little relevance for the isolated, nearly invisible patient suffering from severe CFS/ME.

In the absence of any information about those factors responsible for chronicity, it was good to read "We suggest that the prevalence and impact of severe disease, the pathways to chronicity and to becoming severely affected, and strategies that would benefit such individuals urgently need further study." Given the current vacuum relating to knowledge of the factors leading to chronicity, one is left to wonder about what would be the baseline for 'further' study.

In discussing, "Response to treatment," attention was drawn to the range of effects which a single treatment may produce, noting that in some severely affected cases, treatment may have adverse effects. While emphasising the need for *"…carefully planned research"* it was noted that *"Future studies will need to control for gender, ethnicity, severity, duration, triggering event, co-existent conditions and symptom profile.*" It is difficult to imagine a community which contained enough CFS/ME people to allow for a study in which all seven control factors could be analysed. Such studies would be made more difficult by the absence of information about the cause and progress of the condition being treated.

Without any doubt, the section titled "Therapeutic strategies," is the most controversial section in the report. In the absence of an agreed pathophysiology, it was proposed that psychology-based strategies, graded exercise therapy, cognitive behavioural therapy and pacing were "...*potentially beneficial in modifying the illness.*" No mention was made of studies which had found the proposed treatments of little value or of patient reports which noted that the treatments caused worsening of their symptoms, even though it had been noted in "Ongoing care," that attention should be paid to patient feedback.

However, in apparent recognition that the treatments were not always successful, it was stated "A proportion of patients benefit from more structured specialist approaches, such as graded exercise or cognitive behavioural therapy." An important omission is the lack of information about the size of the proportion which benefitted.

After this wry comment on 'an important omission', there follows a clear and succinct explanation regarding the limited benefit and potentially harmful effects of exercise. This explains why 'pacing', in which the patient is in control, is found helpful by many people who have ME/Ramsay's Disease, while following an externally prescribed, and in some cases, coerced, programme of physical exercise (GET) has been found harmful by the majority.

It needs to be recognised that the benefit of low intensity exercise is that it results in a reduction of blood viscosity, but the level of activity has to be determined by the patient. In contrast, over-activity leads to a change in the shape populations of red blood cells and impaired capillary blood flow. Therefore, the primary problem of the concept of 'graded exercise,' is that it is not known at which level of activity there will be an adverse response, and that level will vary from individual to individual. The observations made in the section, "Graded exercise," need to be considered with this information in mind. So it is not surprising that of one thousand two hundred and fourteen patients studied, six hundred and ten (50%) reported that graded exercise made their condition worse. It was stated "*A successful outcome probably depends on the therapy being initially based on current physical capacity, mutually agreed between the therapist and patient, and adapted according to the physical response.*" But there is no way in which at any particular time a patient can predict his/her response to any level of activity. This implies that any successful outcome was the result of the chance event that the agreed level of activity was within the capacity of the patient.

The section dealing with "Cognitive behavioural therapy," began "Although there is no cure for CFS/ME, the condition has been found to improve in most patients, both with and without treatment: it is good practice to encourage patients to become experts in self-management and to choose between treatment options." With regard to cognitive behavioural therapy it was stated "It involves personal actions – i.e. 'what we do' and 'what we think' – that can affect physiological processes; for example, smoking, excessive alcohol intake and stress can all contribute to illness." In the circumstances where personal actions were considered to determine physiological processes, it was unexpected to find that all three factors which could contribute to illness, share the common feature that they have an adverse effect on the flow properties of blood because they alter blood rheology. Furthermore, the adverse effects on blood rheology would be added to any existing abnormality of the flow properties of the blood CFS/ME patients.

Just as was noted for graded exercise therapy, it was considered that experienced therapists were needed for cognitive behavioural therapy. An indication of the benefits of the therapy is reflected in patients reports in which 67% reported 'no change,' while 26% reported that the treatment made them 'worse.' The disagreement among physicians about the value of graded exercise therapy was repeated with regard to cognitive behavioural therapy. Rather surprisingly it was noted *"The majority of the Working Group accepts that appropriately administered cognitive behavioural therapy can improve functioning in many ambulatory patients with CFS/ME who attend outpatient clinics."* But in order to put that conclusion into perspective it would need to be known what 'many' equates with in percentage terms, and what proportion of the total patient base is able to attend outpatient clinics.

Because of the lack of an accepted cause and pathophysiology of CFS/ME, it was a further surprise to read that "Patients who might benefit can expect to receive a logical explanation of why cognitive behavioural therapy might help them, based on their specific history and principles." In the absence of data, the 'logical explanation,' would be based upon conjecture and guesswork, with the outcome comparable to divining the future by assessing the entrails of a chicken. Thus in a situation in which the availability of some basic information indicated a research need to provide a 'logical explanation,' it was concluded that more research was needed "… to identify which CFS/ME patients derive most benefits from the therapy, etc."

There is no doubt that 'pacing,' or living within the boundaries of physical activity determined by the illness, is the most important factor in determining patient wellbeing. This is reflected in the fact that 89% of two thousand patients considered pacing helpful. As was the case with the other therapies, there was disagreement among physicians about the role of pacing in treatment.

> Many physicians are comfortable with a patient-controlled regime, while others feel a strong need to be imposing an externally-devised treatment programme. Unfortunately it is this latter group which have also controlled policy: hence NICE still recommending a treatment, GET, which will make patients with ME worse.

In contrast to psychology-based therapy, my approach to the treatment of ME people with high values of flat cells in their blood involved three suggestions:

1. With the objective of improving the rate of capillary blood flow, endeavour to increase red blood cell deformability by taking 4grams daily of evening primrose oil; or 6 grams daily of fish oil; or 3 x 400mg tablets of Trental (pentoxifylline)

daily. I do not know which patients will respond to what treatment, and for that reason unless there is recognisable benefit by six weeks, another agent should be tried.

2. Plan a daily pattern of activity, such as walking to the nearest lamp-post and back each day for a week. In the following week walk to the second nearest lamppost for a week. Extend the length of the daily walk on a weekly basis, but walk at your own pace.

3. Do not get involved in arguments – turn your back and walk away. Keep away from stressful events, bearing in mind that such events will worsen your blood flow problem.

For reasons which I will address in the final part of this book, 'cure' is not an option, and the objective is to enable ME people to have a 'normal' – albeit secluded – lifestyle. Many letters and emails have recorded that the suggestions worked. However, cost has been a problem, so it needs to be emphasised that for the oils, the dose levels are the lowest effective doses, so taking 'one to three capsules' as noted on the containers will be a waste of money.

Although "The use of counselling," was discussed, it is not easy to understand how counselling would be of benefit in a condition with a demonstrable problem of blood flow. So it was strange to read that "*Further research is warranted in the form of a larger, randomised, controlled trial to examine the possible benefits of counselling, etc.*" Thus it would seem that the research needs for approaches to therapy were considered to be greater than the need to determine the aetiology and pathophysiology of CFS/ME.

An unexpected aspect of the section, "Symptom control," was that tiredness was not mentioned as a symptom, and symptoms were restricted to sleep problems, mood disturbance and pain.

It is obliquely relevant that in 1970 Ellis et al (56) surveyed the use of vitamin B12 in general practice in the UK, and found that 55.5% of GPs used the vitamin non-specifically for the treatment of tiredness. Three years later, Ellis and Nasser (57) published a paper titled "A pilot study of vitamin B12 in the treatment of tiredness." This involved a double-blind, cross-over trial, of injections of B12 as hydroxocobalamin. Although the effect of the vitamin on tiredness was not discussed specifically, it was concluded "*These results seem to offer support for the widely held belief that vitamin B12 has a definite 'tonic' effect.*" The chance observation on a blood sample from a woman with acute ME, shortly after her GP had given her an injection of hydroxocobalamin, showed there was a marked reduction in the numbers of cup-forms when compared with previous results. In addition there was a marked improvement in wellbeing.

As reported at the Cambridge Symposium, of fourteen pairs of blood samples (pre- and post-B12) provided by GPs, only 50% showed a reduction in cup forms and a loss of symptoms. While it remains unknown why only 50% of cases with acute ME benefited, injections of 1 ml of B12 (as Neocytamen) at 10 to 14 day intervals helped many individuals. This suggested treatment is in accord with the conclusion, "*Specific therapies can be chosen based on advice from relevant guidelines or reviews.*"

An important observation in "Follow-up, transition and recovery," noted that

> *Unfortunately, some patients show little or no response to existing treatment options, and may show no improvement over long periods; while both patient and clinician should continue to review possible ways of improving their situation, the patient should not be made to feel that they are to blame for the lack of response, nor forced into therapies that are inappropriate, unwanted or ineffective for that individual.*

That statement simply recognises the great variability of the way in which the health problems of CFS/ME may present.

> I would want to add that that statement also expresses a degree of respect and compassion for the patient which is distinctly absent in the written and spoken remarks of the Wessely group, and therefore not reflected in many settings, influenced by their views, which purport to provide 'specialist treatment' for CFS/ME.

In addition it was stated "*...the fluctuating nature of CFS/ME means that remissions, setbacks, or more substantial relapses may occur.*" However, while it is recognised that remissions occur in ME, they are not a part of CFS, and there is no recognition of the implications of remissions with regard to the nature of the illness. So it was also unclear why "*A transition represents an opportunity to review the management plans with patients and carers.*"

"Service models" commenced "*Provision of services specifically designed for patients with CFS/ME is either limited or non-existent.*" Because of the relatively low number of cases in any region, the provision of services faces cost-related problems. It was recognised that wherever possible, CFS/ME patients should be managed in their local community. This would involve on-going support for GPs, and for patients and carers. In recognising that

"Dedicated inpatient services for CFS/ME are lacking," there was a need "*...to develop a local network of services to support, in particular, the severely affected, house-bound or bed-bound patients who are currently unable to access services.*"

No comment is offered on Chapter 5, "Children and young people," as this is a field in which I lack experience.

The "Recommendations of the Working Group," were made using five headings:

1) **Recognition and definition of the illness.**

   a) "*The NHS and healthcare professionals should recognise CFS/ME as a chronic illness, etc.*" However, in the USA, CFS is recognised as a collection of disorders, which is in sharp contrast to the concept of ME as a single entity, as defined by Ramsay. Therefore this conclusion will compound the existing confusion concerning nomenclature.

   b) "*...we recommend that the terminology should be reviewed in concert with international work on this topic.*" While this recommendation hits at the very heart of the problem, it has to be a cause for concern that in January 2007 an American group has renamed CFS as ME (myalgic encephalopathy).

2) Treatment and care.

Although the restricted brief of the Working Group meant that it was not required to consider the aetiology and pathogenesis of the problem, it was stated that health care professionals and GPs, "...*should have sufficient awareness, understanding and knowledge of the illness to enable them to recognise, assess, manage and support the patient with CFS/ME.*" But it is puzzling to imagine how a unified concept might develop for a disorder which is characterised by its variability in presenting signs.

Although there was a recognised need for specialists in the disorder, it was unclear where and how specialist training would be given. But the report stated "*Sufficient tertiary-level specialists in CFS/ME should be available to advise and support colleagues in primary and secondary care*" which fails to indicate whether or not specialists will be available.

However, according to the report, patient management should be based upon a partnership with the patient, and should usually extend to the patient's carers and family and be flexible in nature. In general it seems that the road to treatment and care is paved with good intentions, but is this sufficient to help those who are severely ill?

3) Health service planning.

This deals with the need for resources at all levels, and with the need for local authorities to develop the necessary local services. As the provision for services were to be based upon a prevalence of four thousand cases per million of the population, this could lead to local regions with either an over-supply or an undersupply of services.

4) Education and awareness.

While an essential need would be for all healthcare professionals to have adequate education and training, the absence of a unified concept of CFS/ME and the lack of an accepted aetiology and pathophysiology would pose problems for any educational programme.

5) Research.

Although six topics for research were listed, the over-riding importance and significance of the first topic "*Elucidate the aetiology and pathogenesis of CFS/ME,*" indicated that until that research was completed, the relevance of the other topics would remain indeterminable.

Given the restricted nature of its brief, it is not surprising that the Working Group report should have very little to offer those who suffer from ME, or CFS, or CFS/ME, however those disorders are defined. It is possibly tacit recognition of the lightweight nature of the report that led to "Elucidate the aetiology and pathogenesis of CFS/ME" being the first choice for urgent research. To a large extent this is reflected throughout the report where diagnosis, treatment and care recommendations related to an illness of unknown cause with fluctuating variability of symptoms.

From my point of view, it was unfortunate that the Working Group decided, against the evidence, that ME was an entity which had been incorporated into the mix of disorders known as CFS. Given the American interest in the sub-grouping of CFS, it is very likely that the heterogeneous nature of CFS will be revealed in the not too distant future.

This brief, critical summary of the Working Group report fails to match the quality of the criticism contained in "Unhelpful Counsel?" a response dated April 2002, from the Scottish group MERGE (ME Group for Education and Research). The final paragraph of the executive summary read as follows:

In summary, while the Working Group's report may go some way towards improving recognition of the illness, MERGE considers that it has avoided serious consideration of the important issues surrounding the diagnosis and treatment of ME/CFS; that it has given undue emphasis to management strategies of limited applicability; that practical recommendations for social care provisions are lacking; and that, consequently an opportunity to effect real change has been lost.

One can only ponder about the consequences if a different option had followed the discussion on nomenclature (p5):

In recent years CFS has been the preferred medical term for this disorder, or group of disorders, although a large majority of patient support organisations use the term ME. The term ME has been applied to the syndrome – or, according to some interpretations, a subset of it – and is widely used in the community. What would the result have been if the brief had been to review management and practice in the field of ME?

It should be noted that other groups have also expressed concern about the contents of the Working Group's report, although it should be recognised that the Group was hamstrung by the very restrictive nature of its brief.

The Canadian Guidelines

These comments on the so-called "Canadian Guidelines" are derived from the 2005 publication by Carruthers and van de Sande, titled "Myalgic encephalomyelitis/chronic fatigue syndrome: a clinical case definition and guidelines for medical practitioners: An overview of the Canadian Consensus document." The original report was published as a one-hundred-and-eight-page paper in the Journal of Chronic Fatigue Syndrome in 2003.

The list of contributors/authors of the Consensus document includes several well-known investigators who have been studying various aspects of CFS for a long time and published many papers on the topic. But no published work has identified a cause for CFS, or explained the pathophysiology of the disorder. While the document claimed to be a consensus, subsequent publications by some of the participants do not reveal a change in their (varying) concepts.

Given that the study was Canadian in origin, it is surprising that probably the best known Canadian investigator in the field of ME, Dr. Byron Hyde, was not a member of the group.

The nomenclature used was puzzling. Even though Ramsay's work was cited, there is little in the document which would indicate that his views had any bearing on the topic. In addition, the fact that most, if not all of the American workers would have been studying CFS, which is recognised as a heterogeneous disorder needing to be sub-grouped, it is difficult to understand why it was stated in the introduction *"Myalgic encephalomyelitis, and chronic fatigue syndrome are used interchangeably and this illness is referred to as ME/CFS."* This is such a radical step (as it rejects Ramsay's criteria out of hand, and it rejects what has been published concerning the unitary nature of ME) that some explanation for synthesising two very different disorders might have been expected, but it was simply stated as fact.

So at the very outset, an obstacle to obtaining an understanding of ME has been created which persisted throughout the report and the relevance of the Consensus became debateable. While the Expert Consensus Panel approved of ME and CFS being used inter-changeably, such a proposal would be unacceptable to many investigators. In his contribution to the Chief Medical Officer's Working Group, Dr. Hyde stated quite unambiguously that ME and CFS were different disorders. Given the time that he has worked in the field of ME, it was surprising to find a dearth of publications on the topic. A PubMed search for "Hyde BM" revealed that he was the joint author of six papers unrelated to ME, but in 1991 he had published a paper titled, "Myalgic encephalomyelitis(chronic fatigue syndrome): an historical perspective." Yet in the book which was based on the 1990 Cambridge Symposium on ME, Hyde, Goldstein and Levine wrote about ME/CFS, and the title of my contribution concerning ME was changed to ME/CFS.

Perhaps, because it was possible to diagnose ME prior to the release of CFS in 1988, ME organisations persist in several countries, and CFS is recognised as a collection of different disorders. Even before the release in 1994 by Fukuda et al of wider criteria for CFS, it was recognised that CFS was not a single disorder as, for example, in 1992, Levine noted, *"One useful aspect of international working groups could be the development of improved guidelines to sub-classify CFS using sub-groups such as those with or without documented immune dysfunction, etc."*

Since 1992, many others have proposed a need for sub-grouping CFS, so the concept of a single diagnosis, ME, being interchangeable with the multifaceted CFS, has to be a potential source of confusion. Furthermore, in material published by American experts since the 2003 publication of the Consensus, there is nothing to indicate that their approach to CFS has changed along the lines reported in that document. This situation could indicate that "consensus" might have been a "lack of stated objections".

In the discussion titled "Etiology," a role for infective triggers is noted, followed by comment on indications of immune dysfunction. While *"other prodromal events,"* such as immunisation, anaesthetics, physical trauma, exposure to environmental pollutants, chemicals and heavy metals were noted, there was no discussion about how such diverse events related to infective triggers or to immune dysfunction, or how they might function as a trigger.

The point is that all such factors induce change in the internal environment, and may stimulate changes in the shape populations of red blood cells, potentiating problems in the flow properties of blood. So it is very relevant that two important contributors to the

Consensus meeting had been informed of this. During a visit to Ottawa I met Ms Neilson, and she attended my illustrated presentation in which I showed the red cell changes in ME and other chronic disorders, and emphasised the adverse effects of such cells on the rate of capillary blood flow. On May 11, 1996, my daily diary records that I had evening meal with Dr. Carruthers, which was followed by a long discussion. In fact, we were the last to leave the restaurant. This implies that my published findings were simply rejected, rather than being unknown.

Under "Epidemiology," it was stated *"Relapses can occur several years after remission,"* which is the only time the term remission appears in the publication. Remissions are a key feature of ME, but their occurrence creates a problem for those who consider that a persistent viral infection, or an ongoing immunological abnormality, is a key feature in the pathophysiology. Possibly for this reason, only very rarely are remissions discussed or even mentioned. But unless any proposed natural history can account for remissions, it has to be rejected.

Given the make-up of the Consensus Panel, it is not surprising that "The clinical working case definition of ME/CFS" was structured in a manner similar to that of the 1994 CDC criteria and the "Symptoms and signs" were discussed sequentially. Fatigue was the primary interest, and there was no mention of tiredness which is the term used by ME people in other countries to describe their problem. An unrecognised problem of the term fatigue is that the dictionary definition considers fatigue to be the result from long-continued exertion, but ME people do not need to run up stairs to become tired. The term 'post-exertional malaise/or fatigue' was used in preference to Ramsay's term of muscle fatigability. Sir John Ellis had drawn attention in 1970 to the fact that patients did not use the terms fatigue or malaise, which he considered were textbook terms. However, it was noted that post-exertional malaise and fatigue was observed to occur with *"...a tendency for other associated symptoms within the cluster of symptoms, to worsen,"* and a slow recovery period was noted.

Possible causes of the effects of exertion were not discussed, even though in 1992, in the book by Hyde et al, both Dr. Mena and Dr. Goldstein had noted that post-exercise SPECT scans showed a greater reduction in regional cerebral blood flow than in the pre-exercise scan.

Physical activity in excess of some undefined level induces changes in the shape populations of red blood cells. In 1993 we reported the effects on red cell shape of inducing trigger finger fatigue in ME people and in healthy controls. The results were consistent with the reported SPECT results of physical activity on regional cerebral blood flow. In post-race blood samples from marathon runners, increased numbers of cup forms have been found. So it is very likely that post-exertional malaise reflects the adverse effects of shape-changed, poorly deformable red cells on capillary blood flow, with inadequate rates of delivery of oxygen and nutrient substrates to sustain normal tissue function. Because reduced rates of cerebral blood flow will lead to brain dysfunction, this could explain the sleep problems and the neurological/cognitive manifestations of the disorder.

"Symptoms and signs" were discussed under five headings of which 'fatigue' was the first and considered to be "...*an inappropriate label*." Even though tiredness is the term favoured by ME people it was not listed as an alternative. It could be relevant that physiologists interpret muscle fatigue in terms of poor blood flow leading to oxygen insufficiency, so it is possible that what is experienced as fatigue is simply a manifestation of a systemic problem of blood flow.

A discussion of 'sleep dysfunction' gave no consideration to the possibility that the changes in regional cerebral blood flow shown by SPECT might result in sleep disturbance, yet it would be surprising if the brain would continue to function normally when the rate of blood flow was reduced.

In the section on 'pain' it was stated *"The chronic pain is thought to be due to a dysfunction of the pain processing areas of the central nervous system."* The possibility that the 'dysfunction' might be due to a hypoxic state because of impaired capillary blood flow arose from studies in another disorder.

I received a request to assess anonymous blood samples from people with the whole body pain problem of arachnoiditis. Blood samples were duly received, processed and assessed and showed the common feature of high values for flat cells. The routine result sheet included a copy of the micrograph of red cells, the percentages of cell classes compared with control values, and where appropriate, a suggestion that 4 grams daily of evening primrose oil might prove beneficial. Subsequently, I received a note from the organiser to say that she had been told that some of the people concerned had reported that after taking evening primrose oil, their pain levels were reduced greatly. As the evening primrose oil would improve capillary blood flow and oxygen delivery, the reduction in pain might have been due to the correction of a hypoxic state. However, shortly after, the organiser died and no further work was done with arachnoiditis. Fibromyalgia is another whole body pain problem, and it is noteworthy that blood samples from six hundred and twenty-three cases had high values for flat cells as was found in arachnoiditis, but I have not had an opportunity to do further work with fibromyalgia.

The discussion of 'neurological/cognitive manifestations' noted that PET scans revealed a decreased rate of glucose metabolism and that SPECT scans, "...*reveal significantly lower cortical/cerebellar regional cerebral blood flow*" in various parts of the brain, which "...*may play a role in cognitive impairment and activity limitations.*" There was no comment about the possibility that a "...*decreased rate of glucose metabolism*" would be expected if the rate of blood flow was reduced, and a reluctance to accept the importance of normal rates of blood flow to sustain normal tissue function was reflected in the statement that reduced blood flow "...***may** play a role in cognitive impairment, etc.*" In his study of ME people by SPET, Costa reported not only a reduction in blood flow rates in the brainstem, but also a generalised reduction in brain perfusion. In other disorders with changed red cell shape populations, SPECT scans show reduced rates of regional cerebral blood flow in different regions of the brain. The cognitive effects of reduced cerebral blood flow (as shown by xenon inhalation) were observed in patients with Huntington's Disease, by Tanahashi et al in 1985. While the irreversible punctuate lesions observed by MRI could be demonstrating the presence of focal ischaemic necrosis resulting from capillary blockage by stiff red cells, temporary areas of brightness could be due to the increased transudation resulting from an increase in intra-capillary pressure needed to overcome the resistance to flow of poorly deformable red cells. Such demonstrations of impaired cerebral blood flow provide a basis for understanding how 'brain fog' might develop with its attendant cognitive problems.

In "Other symptoms," it was stated that in addition to other eye problems, "blurred or double vision" had been noted.

It is probably relevant that when ME people came to visit me, they had to walk up three flights of stairs to my office. I always shook hands in order to determine if they had cold hands, then asked "When you got to the top of the stairs, did you notice any changes in vision?" Almost all had cold hands and reported blurred vision, so I would tell them, "You have a blood flow problem, come in and we will talk about it." Subsequent red cell shape analysis of a blood sample revealed changed red cell shape populations.

Although much was written about "autonomic manifestations", in the terms of Ramsay's criteria, dysautonomia would have excluded a diagnosis of ME – but if there were a systemic problem of blood flow it could be anticipated that capillary blood flow in the nerves of the autonomic nervous system would be impaired.

Several different aspects of the 'neuro-endocrine manifestations' were discussed, without recognition of the need for normal rates of blood flow to sustain normal function of nerve tissue and endocrine glands. As secreting glands are particularly sensitive to deprivation of their metabolic needs, it could be anticipated that gland dysfunction would result when the rate of capillary blood flow was impaired. It could be speculated that the identity and nature of the dysfunction would be related to poorer cerebral blood flow in specific regions. For example, it was stated, *"Hypothalamic/pituitary/adrenal axis and autonomic nervous system dysregulation may lessen patients' adaptability to stressful and overload situations. Stress may cause disorientation, anxiety, worsening of other symptoms and trigger a 'crash'."* It was demonstrated in 1975 that the stress hormones stiffen red blood cells, exacerbating any existing change in the red cell shape population, so the adverse effects on capillary blood flow provide a basis for understanding the pathophysiology of such events and why they lead to a relapse.

The section 'immune manifestations' recognised that many infectious agents trigger ME/CFS and some of these are discussed. But no mention was made of the English claims relating to enteroviruses. While there was much speculation about various factors, there was the puzzling statement, *"The elevated levels of many intracellular pathogens, suggest that immune dysfunction plays a primary role."* But if the pathogens were intracellular, they would be sheltered from the immune response. As it was noted that elevated levels of immunoglobulins had been reported, there would be a concomitant change in the internal environment, stimulating change in the shape populations of red cells. This has been found to happen in a healthy subject after immunisation. But there is no recognition of the fact that the stimulation of the immune system does more than induce changes in the system, yet the final sentence stated *"Physical exercise and overload situations may trigger or exacerbate immune symptoms.*" The significant point is that physical activity changes the shape population of red cells, which will be additive to those relating to the status of any immune response. Nothing in the section provides an explanation for how immune dysfunction is related causally to fatigue or to other dysfunctional systems.

The 'clinical evaluation of ME/CFS' has the objectives of recognising the characteristic features of ME/CFS (evidently as a single entity) and excluding alternative diagnoses, which does not differ greatly from Ramsay's approach. While there is a considerable degree of agreement in the approach to clinical evaluation with that of the Australian Guidelines which dealt with CFS, the Consensus document deals with ME/CFS. What is different is the extent of the 'additional testing' in the 'laboratory and investigations protocol', none of which were used by Ramsay and others to diagnose ME. Although it was noted that SPECT scans would be performed, 'if indicated', there was no comment about what situations would indicate a need for a SPECT scan. The extent of the testing procedures was so great (21 tests listed) that it is difficult to consider the objective of the tests was to confirm or reject a decision reached by differential diagnosis. However, by ignoring the fact that remissions occur, the opportunity to determine if the altered values return to normal is lost. Yet red cell shape analysis of blood samples taken during remissions revealed normal results.

In 2004, Jason et al (58) published a paper titled, "Comparing the Fukuda et al criteria and the Canadian case definition for Chronic Fatigue Syndrome," and the abstract commenced:

> *Because the pathogenesis of Chronic Fatigue Syndrome (CFS) has yet to be determined, case definitions have relied on clinical observations in classifying signs and symptoms for diagnosis. The selection of diagnostic signs and symptoms has major implications for which individuals are diagnosed with CFS and how seriously the illness is viewed by health care providers, disability insurers and rehabilitation planners, and patients and their families and friends.*

This is clearly written in the American idiom concerning CFS with no relevance to ME. While it is true that the nature of a diagnosis will impact on patients in many ways, it seems reasonable to ask to what extent are symptoms valid criteria? When many symptoms are present, involving different physiological systems, is it being proposed that each symptom has its own pathophysiology? Or is it more reasonable to propose, as has been suggested, that the variety of symptoms arises from the single factor of impaired blood flow, with the location of symptoms reflecting regions with more severe impedance to blood flow due to the random distribution of small capillaries?

The study by Jason et al (58) involved twenty-three cases who met the Canadian criteria for ME/CFS; twelve cases who met the Fukuda criteria for CFS; and thirty-three in a chronic fatigue-psychiatric group. Statistical analysis of the frequency of the symptoms reported by each participant showed that there were differences amongst the three groups. It was concluded

> *The findings suggest that both the Canadian and Fukuda et al case definitions select individuals who are statistically significantly different from psychiatric*

controls with chronic fatigue, with the Canadian criteria selecting cases with Dr.
Simpsons psychiatric co-morbidity, more physical functional impairment and more
fatigue/weakness, neuropsychiatric and neurological symptoms.

Given the small sample sizes, the relevance of these findings is unclear. Maybe the differences relate to the inclusive nature of the Fukuda et al criteria for CFS involving different disorders, enhanced by the Canadian belief that ME and CFS are interchangeable terms.

From an ME viewpoint, a problem with such a study is the assumption that at any point in time, the well-being of all patients in any group is the same, when in fact it is known to alter from hour to hour – quite apart from remissions. To some extent this time-related variability may be reflected in a postscript, 'Notes,' where it was stated that only 65.2% of participants diagnosed with the Canadian case definition endorsed the term 'post-exertional malaise', and that 78.2% indicated the presence of memory and concentration problems. Such values seem to indicate that the Canadian case definition had failed to select a uniform group for study.

'Treatment guidelines' were considered under the headings, 'Self-help strategies,' 'Self-empowered exercise,' and 'Symptom management and treatment.' With the objective of supporting the patient, it was stated, *"Reduce the patient's confusion with a positive diagnosis, reassure continuing care, and give realistic hope."* Patients were encouraged *"...to be as active as possible without aggravating symptoms, and then encourage him/her to gradually extend boundaries at his/her **own pace, and as able**"* (my emphasis). Such good advice emphasises the need for the opinions of patients, concerning their level of well-being, to be recognised.

Under the sub-heading 'Guidelines,' it was noted that because the treating physician knows the patient best, *"...he should co-ordinate treatment and rehabilitation."* Unless this was the author's way of saying that ME/CFS has an organic basis, it is unclear what is meant by *"The biological pathophysiology of ME/CFS is a reality that must be respected, etc."* Patients were to be involved in setting realistic goals, although given the fluctuating nature of the symptoms, setting a realistic goal may not be a simple matter for the patient.

Under the heading 'Self-help strategies' there are two puzzling statements. After commenting on the relevance of cognitive behaviour therapy, it was stated, *"Proponents ignore the documented pathophysiology of ME/CFS, disregard the reality of the patients' symptoms, etc.,"* and *"Some physicians, who are cognizant of the biological pathophysiology of ME/CFS, teach patients coping skills, etc."* But there is no documented pathophysiology for ME/CFS, and the statements contrast with that of Jason et al, (57) *"Because the pathogenesis of Chronic Fatigue Syndrome has yet to be determined, etc."* However, the recommended strategies provide a wide range of common sense suggestions for a restricted lifestyle, although the basis for the need for nutritional supplements is arguable.

Several important observations are made in the section 'Self-powered exercise' one of which is that *"...patients are often prescribed exercise unwisely."* Here, in Dunedin, ME people responded positively to exercise performed in a hot pool, standing shoulder deep. It was assumed that the buoyancy of the water greatly reduced the level of the muscle energy expended doing callisthenics. So it was rather surprising that the use of warm pools was not mentioned.

An important conclusion stated, "It is imperative for them (patients) to maintain autonomy over the intensity and pacing of exercise and activities." This view was reinforced in the statement, "Externally paced 'Graded Exercise Programs', or programs based on the premise that patients are misperceiving their activity limits or illness **must be avoided**."

It was stated, "Significantly impaired oxygen consumption levels suggest there may be an abnormal reliance on anaerobic energy pathways during exercise in patients with ME/CFS, thus exercises that would be aerobic for healthy individuals may be anaerobic for patients." But when shape-changed, poorly deformable red cells impede blood flow in the microcirculation, what is noted as "impaired oxygen consumption levels," could be due to an inadequate rate of oxygen delivery, manifested as an effect of reduced rates of capillary blood flow plus the reduced rates of release of oxygen from shape-changed red cells.

> The paragraph above sets out what I believe to be one of the most central, important facts concerning Ramsay's Disease (ME): If we assume that the 'impaired blood flow' in muscles, which can be accounted for by the shape-changed red blood cell population, causes the failure of the aerobic muscle metabolism, leading to immediate use of the anaerobic muscle metabolism, this would explain how a minimum physical effort can produce tiredness (fatigue) comparable to that produced by extreme exertion in a normally functioning muscle. It would also explain the development of pain caused by immediate build-up of waste products (lactic acid) in muscles, and the delayed and prolonged period of recovery from apparently minimal exertion.
>
> Under these conditions, it is evident that any form of exercise which is imposed beyond the narrow limits created by the nature of the illness will be damaging – equivalent to the imposition of extreme and protracted hard labour on a normal person. Refusal, and strong emotional reactions against such 'treatment', becomes perfectly reasonable and understandable. People who have ME are justified in their protests against Graded Exercise Therapy.

'Symptom management and treatment' has the apparent objective of improving patient well-being, and it was stated that *"No pharmaceutical is universally effective."* This was followed by the sound advice *"Keep regime as simple, safe, effective, and as inexpensive as possible."* Perhaps a major omission was the lack of reference to the need for treatment (if any) during remissions, which may be brief or prolonged.

Symptom management was discussed under seven headings; sleep disturbances, pain, fatigue, cognitive manifestations, autonomic manifestations, neuroendocrine manifestations, immune manifestations. It was rather peculiar to find recommendations for complementary therapies such as aromatherapy, magnetic pulsers, Bio-Resonance therapy, and biofeedback, in a consensus document which implies agreement from all members of the panel. As physiology texts consider that muscle fatigue is a consequence of inadequate oxygen availability due to insufficient blood flow, it is difficult to understand how fatigue might be relieved by such remedies as, *"…restorative resting postures, massage therapy, craniosacral therapy and aromatherapy.*" Is it reasonable to suggest that experienced investigators such as Professor Klimas and Professor De Meirleir would recommend such treatments?

Among the pharmaceuticals listed, vitamin B12 as cyanocobalamin was suggested with the note, "Anecdotal reports and studies suggest some ME/CFS patients with normal blood counts improve in energy level, cognitive ability, weakness and mood with mega dose B12 injections, etc." In my presentation to the Cambridge Symposium on ME in 1990, I reported that injections of B12 as hydroxocobalamin in patients with acute ME reduced symptom severity and reduced the numbers of cup-transformed red cells. An unexplained aspect was that the benefits of 1ml of Neocytamen at ten to fourteen day intervals were effective in only 50% of cases and there was no response in the other 50%. But this observation draws attention to the fact that none of the seventy odd papers in the 1992 book on ME/CFS by Hyde, Goldstein and Levine are included in the fifty-one cited references.

While it is not known if other members of the cobalamin family have beneficial effects, a Canadian physician emailed me for the address of the makers of Neocytamen. Evidently he procured the vitamin, as several weeks later he wrote to me on February 6, 1997 as follows:

> *I thought you would be pleased with a very brief report on a patient I first began to see in December 1994, having suffered from chronic pain and depression. There were ample reasons in her history to account for this because of a series of misfortunes. In any event, I started her on a treatment program, and although there was substantial improvement, it was only after she had a test dose of vitamin B12 1mg injection, that within the next forty-eight hours she was very much improved. By this time she had been diagnosed as having fibromyalgia.*
>
> *When I saw her today, February 5th, she had been taking B12 injections twice a week and there was a major improvement. She is now free of pain, can walk without pain, can move her arms freely, and she reports that she now thinks she is almost back to where she was before she became ill in the first place. She is taking, in addition to her B12 injections, niacin 500mg TID, vitamin E 1200iu per day, pantothenic acid 1 g TID and selenium 200mcg OD. However, this major improvement came almost immediately after the first injection of vitamin B12.*

In the sections, 'cognitive manifestations, autonomic manifestations and neuroendocrine manifestations,' there was no recognition of the implications of the reductions in regional cerebral blood flow which had been demonstrated by SPECT scans. Yet it seems illogical to consider that normal brain function would continue if cerebral blood flow was reduced. This matter becomes more focussed in the section 'neuroendocrine manifestations' where depression is discussed without reference to the literature concerning SPECT studies in subjects suffering from depressive illness. In those studies, a direct association of depression and reduced regional blood flow has been reported, and regions with reduced blood flow during depression were shown to have normal rates of blood flow after the resolution of the depression.

As immunization was discussed, it is very relevant that during an active immune response the change in the internal environment is sufficient to change the shape populations of red cells. In a healthy subject there was an immediate post-vaccination increase in cells with altered margins which persisted for four weeks, accompanied by a very slight malaise. Therefore it could be expected that vaccination of a subject with ME/CFS would be followed by a relapse.

In a concluding section it was stated, "*Great strides have been made in the knowledge about ME/CFS in the last decade*" but it is likely that the authors of most of the published material would not have accepted the proposal that ME and CFS were interchangeable terms. Nor is there evidence that participation in the Consensus has changed the opinions of participants. For example, in the preface to the report of an Australian meeting in 2005, Professor De Meirleir was quoted as follows: "*Myalgic encephalomyelitis/chronic fatigue syndrome is a chronic, low grade inflammatory disorder, with a defective immune system at the level of the gut and blood brain barrier. It represents an immune-vigilance disorder with low grade sepsis.*" Such a concept is so radically different from the findings of Ramsay and others in ME, and totally different from the Canadian Consensus that it is timely to introduce the name "Ramsay's Disease (ME)," with the objective of reducing the confusion. Furthermore, the introduction to the report stated "*The Adelaide ME/CFS Forum was an informal meeting of researchers and clinicians invited to present their work and reach consensus around clinical, diagnostic and research criteria for ME/CFS.*" In sharp contrast to the statement by Professor De Meirleir, but with an equally controversial approach it was stated:

> *ME/CFS is a broad diagnosis which includes a spectrum of clinical syndromes linked to known infectious agents including Ross River virus, Epstein Barr virus, Q Fever, Lyme disease, parvovirus B19, and toxic exposures such as organophosphates. These syndromes are characterised by neurological, gastrointestinal, cardiovascular and myoarthralgic features. Severe forms can present with paresis, seizures, intractable savage headache and life-threatening complications. The re-naming to chronic fatigue syndrome in 1988, giving misplaced emphasis to 'fatigue' trivialises the substantial disability of ME/CFS which can extend to the patient being wheelchair or bed-bound, requiring 24 hour care.*

Given the expressed antipathy to 'CFS' the question arises why is the topic titled ME/CFS? In a 'Forum Review', Dr. M. Barratt stated, "*Professor De Meirleir presented an epitome of over 5000 research papers on the topic since 1999*", but despite this evidence of research interest, there is no accepted cause or pathophysiology for the disorder. Such a situation implies that for one reason or another, investigators are following the wrong leads and/or inappropriate concepts.

So how is the Consensus document to be evaluated? After all, it is more than twenty-five years since I met my first ME patient and twenty-one years since our first report concerning the changed flow properties of ME blood. But the subsequent publication of other abnormal features of ME blood, and the implications of reports from neuroimaging studies showing reduced regional cerebral blood flow, failed to gain recognition from the Consensus panel. Given that many of the Americans on the panel would have considered CFS in terms of the Fukuda et al criteria, and lack any knowledge of the published work on ME, it is surprising that there was a consensus about using the terms 'ME' and 'CFS' interchangeably. Despite the preference for ME, there was only one mention of remissions, which are a characteristic feature of ME. **The significance of remissions is the constraints they apply to any postulated aetiopathology which must be able to account for the switch from being unwell to being well, as distinct from relapses which may involve a shift from being unwell to being very unwell.** Just what disorder the Consensus guidelines were defining is unclear, as the Jason et al study (58) noted that only 65% endorsed 'post-exertional malaise' as a problem, yet this is a key factor in Ramsay's criteria. On the other hand, the Consensus draws attention to the need for patients to control their physical activity and the need to avoid Graded Exercise Programmes and to retain autonomy over what they are able to do. While Ramsay considered that in ME, the usual laboratory tests would be normal, the Consensus lists no fewer than 21 test procedures, although there was no detailed account of the utility of the tests. It is difficult to escape the conclusion that the Consensus guidelines were formulated by a panel in which members agreed not to disagree, rather than reach a consensus.

So the question arises, what benefits for sufferers can be derived from the results of the time and effort put into the production of the three guidelines? The answer is, probably not very many, if any. Much mental effort has been put into the production of the Australian Guidelines, the CMO's Working Group and the Canadian Consensus Panel, but has this expenditure of time and money been productive? Where the Australians worked with CFS, the CMO's Working Group rejected ME as an entity and used CFS/ME, while the Canadians adopted the view that ME and CFS were terms which could be used interchangeably. Because of the use of three different names for the topic, the chief question would be "If different entities are being discussed, is there any reason to think that the results from their investigations should be similar?"

While their conclusions were not greatly disparate, neither the Australian nor the Canadian groups gave recognition to the possibility that changes in the flow properties of the blood might be the primary factor. In contrast, the Working Group was clearly hindered by the restrictive nature of its brief. None of the three groups recognised an aetiopathology which might have provided some objectivity to their discussions, but it is clear that until an appropriate aetiopathology is developed no substantial progress concerning management and treatment can be expected. This conclusion is reflected in the CMO's Working Group's recommendation for research, the first of which was to, *"Elucidate the aetiology and pathogenesis of CFS/ME."* Evidently the recommendation carried little weight as the Medical Research Council has funded research in the bio-psychosocial field but no research has been funded to explore the biomedical model.

Chapter IV References

1. Holmes GP, Kaplan JE, Gantz NM, et al. Chronic fatigue syndrome: a working case definition. Ann Intern Med 1988; 108:387-9.
2. Strauss SE, Tosato G, Armstrong G, et al. Persisting fatigue in adults with evidence of Epstein-Barr virus infection. Ann Intern Med 1985; 103:7-16.
3. Archard LC, Bowles NE, Behan PO, et al. Postviral fatigue syndrome: persistence of enterovirus RNA in muscle and elevated creatine kinase. J Roy Soc Med 1988; 81:326-9.
4. Manu P, Lane TJ, Matthews DA. The frequency of the chronic fatigue syndrome in patients with symptoms of persistent fatigue. Ann Intern Med 1988; 109:554-6.
5. Lloyd AR, Wakefield D, Broughton CR, et al. What is myalgic encephalomyelitis? Lancet 1988;i: 1286-7.(Letter)
6. Ramsay AM. Myalgic encephalomyelitis or what? Lancet 1988;ii: 100. (Letter)
7. David As, Wessely S, Pelosi AJ, et al. Myalgic encephalomyelitis or what? Lancet 1988;ii: 100-1. (Letter)
8. Lloyd AR, Hickie I, Broughton CR, et al. Prevalence of chronic fatigue syndrome in an Australian population. Med J Aust 1990; 153:522-8.
9. Sharpe MC, Archard LC, Banatvala JE, et al. A report – chronic fatigue syndrome: guidelines for research. J Roy Soc Med 1991; 84:118-21.
10. Krupp LB, Mendelson WB, Friedman K. An overview of chronic fatigue syndrome. J Clin Psychiatry 1991; 52:403-10.
11. Lane TJ, Manu P, Matthews DA. Depression and somatisation in the chronic fatigue syndrome. Am J Med 1991; 91:335-44.
12. Manu P, Lane TJ, Matthews DA. Chronic fatigue and chronic fatigue syndrome: clinical, epidemiology and aetiological classification. Ciba Foundation Symposium 1993; 173:23-31.
13. Schluederberg A, Strauss SE, Peterson P, et al. NIH Conference. Chronic fatigue syndrome research. Definition and medical outcome assessment. Ann Intern Med 1992; 117:325-31.
14. Levine PH. Epidemiologic aspects of chronic fatigue syndrome/myalgic encephalomyelitis. In : Hyde BM, Goldstein J, Levine PH (eds); The clinical and scientific basis of myalgic encephalomyelitis/chronic fatigue syndrome. The Nightingale Research Foundation, Ottawa, 1992, pp196-205.
15. Bates DW, Schmitt W, Buchwald D, et al. Prevalence of fatigue and chronic fatigue syndrome in a primary care practice. Arch Intern Med 1993; 153:2759-65.
16. Bates DW, Buchwald D, Lee J, et al. A comparison of case definitions of chronic fatigue syndromes. Clin Infect Dis 1994; 18 (Suppl 1): S11-5.
17. Fukuda K, Strauss SE, Hickie I, et al. The chronic fatigue syndrome: a comprehensive approach to its definition and study. International Chronic Fatigue Syndrome Study Group. Ann Intern Med 1994; 121: 953-9.
18. Buchwald D, Umali P, Umali J, et al. Chronic fatigue and chronic fatigue syndrome: prevalence in a Northwest healthcare system. Ann Intern Med 1995; 123:81-8.

19. Wessely S, Chalder T, Hirsch S, et al. Psychological symptoms, somatic symptoms, and psychiatric disorder in chronic fatigue and chronic fatigue syndrome: a prospective study in primary care. Am J Psychiatry 1996; 153:1050-9.
20. Komaroff AL, Fagioli LR, Geiger AM, et al. An examination of the working case definition of chronic fatigue syndrome. Am J Med 1995; 100:56-64.
21. Simpson LO, Shand BI, Olds RJ, et al. Red cell and haemorheological changes in multiple sclerosis. Pathology 1987; 19:51-5.
22. Swank RL. Subcutaneous haemorrhages in multiple sclerosis. Neurology 1958; 8:497-8.
23. Swank RL, Roth JC, Woody DC. Cerebral blood flow and red cell delivery in normal subjects and in multiple sclerosis. Neurol Res 1983; 5:37-59.
24. Kury PG, Ramwell PW, McConnell HM. The effects of prostaglandin E1 and E2 on the human erythrocyte as monitored by spin labels. Biochim Biophys Res Commun 1974; 56:478-83.
25. Rasmussen H, Lake W, Allen JE. The effects of catecholamines and prostaglandins upon human and rat erythrocytes. Biochim Biophys Acta 1975; 411:63-73.
26. Simpson LO. Red cell shape in multiple sclerosis. NZ Med J 1992; 105:136.(Letter)
27. Sackheim HA, Prohovnik I, Moeller JR, et al. Regional cerebral blood flow in mood disorders. 1. Comparison of major depression and normal controls at rest. Arch Gen Psychiatry 1990; 47:60-70.
28. Sackheim HA, Prohovnik I. Moeller JR, et al. Regional cerebral blood flow in mood disorders. 2. Comparison of major depression and Alzheimer's disease. J Nucl Med 1993; 34:1090-101.
29. Nobler MS, Sackheim HA, Prohovnik I, et al. Regional cerebral blood flow in mood disorders. 3. Treatment and clinical response. Arch Gen Psychiatry 1994; 51:884-97.
30. Rubin E, Sackheim HA, Prohovnik I, et al. Regional cerebral blood flow in mood disorders. 4. Comparison of mania and depression. Psychiatry Res 1995; 61:1-10.
31. Nobler MS, Roose P, Prohovnik I, et al. Regional cerebral blood flow in mood disorders. 5. Effects of antidepressant medication in late-life depression. Am J Geriatr Psychiatry 2000; 8:289-96.
32. Bench CJ, Friston KJ, Brown RG, et al. The anatomy of melancholia – focal abnormalities of cerebral blood flow in major depression. Psychol Med 1992; 22:607-15.
33. Dolan RJ, Bench CJ, Brown RG, et al. Regional cerebral blood flow abnormalities in depressed patients with cognitive impairment. J Neurol Neurosurg Psychiatry 1992; 55:768-83.
34. Lucey JV, Costa DC, Adshead G, et al. Brain blood flow in anxiety disorders: OCD, panic disorder with agoraphobia and post-traumatic stress disorder. Br J Psychiatry 1997; 171:346-50.

35. Dolan RJ, Bench CJ, Brown RG, et al. Neuropsychological dysfunction in depression: the relationship to regional cerebral blood flow. Psychol Med 1994; 24:849-57.

36. Bench CJ, Friston KJ, Brown RG, et al. Regional cerebral blood flow in depression measured by positron emission tomography: the relationship with clinical dimensions. Psychol Med 1993; 23:579-90.

37. Bench CJ, Frackowiak RS, Dolan RJ. Changes in regional cerebral blood flow on recovery from depression. Psychol Med 1995; 25:247-61.

38. O'Connell RA, Sireci SN jnr, Fastov ME, et al. The role of SPECT brain imaging in assessing psychopathology in the medically ill. Gen Hosp Psychiatry 1991; 13:305-12.

39. Austin MP, Dougall N, Ross M, et al. Single photon emission tomography with 99mTC-exametazime in major depression and the pattern of brain activity underlying the psychotic/neurotic continuum. J Affect Disord 1992; 26:31-43.

40. Schwartz RB, Komaroff AL, Garada BM, et al. SPECT imaging of the brain: comparison of findings in patients with chronic fatigue syndrome, AIDS Dementia Complex and unipolar depression. Am J Roentgenol 1994; 162:943-51.

41. Fischler B, D'Haenen H, Cluydts R, et al. Comparison of 99mTCHMPAO SPECT scans between chronic fatigue, major depression and healthy controls: an exploratory study of regional cerebral blood flow. Neuropsychobiology 1996; 34:175-83.

42. Perico CA, Skaf CR, Yamada A, et al. Relationships between regional cerebral blood flow and separate symptom clusters of major depression: a single photon emission computed tomography study using statistical parametric mapping. Neurosci Letters 2005; 384:265-70.

43. Simpson LO. Chronic tiredness and idiopathic chronic fatigue – a connection? NJ Med 1992:80:211-6.

44. Kamada T, Yamashita T, Baba Y, et al. Dietary sardine oil increases erythrocyte membrane fluidity in diabetic patients. Diabetes 1986; 35:604-11.

45. Simpson LO. Myalgic encephalomyelitis (ME): a haemorheological disorder manifested as impaired capillary blood flow. J Orthomol Med 1997; 12:69-76.

46. Simpson LO, Herbison GP. The results from red cell shape analyses of blood sampLes from members of myalgic encephalomyelitis organisations in 4 countries. J Orthomol Med 1997; 12:221-6.

47. Simpson LO, O'Neill DJ. Red blood cell shape, symptoms and reportedly helpful treatments in Americans with chronic disorders. J Orthomol Med 2001; 16:157-65.

48. Simpson LO, O'Neill DJ. Red blood cell shapes in women with fibromyalgia and the implication for capillary blood flow and tissue function. J Orthomol Med 2001; 16:197-204.

49. Simpson LO. On the pathophysiology of ME/CFS. NZ Fam Phys 2002; 29:426-7.

50. Working Group RACP. Chronic fatigue syndrome clinical practice guidelines – 2002. Med J Aust 2002; 176(9 suppl): S17-55.

51. Simpson LO, Murdoch JC, Herbison GP. Red cell shape changes following trigger finger fatigue in subjects with chronic tiredness and healthy controls. NZ Med J 1993; 106:104-7.

52. Markesbery WR, Butterfield DA. A scanning electron microscope study of erythrocytes in Huntington's Disease. Biochim Biophys Res Commun 1977; 78:560-4.

53. Tanahashi N, Meyer JS, Ishikawa Y, et al. Cerebral blood flow and cognitive testing correlate in Huntington's Disease. Arch Neurol 1985; 42:1169-75.

54. Ajmani RS, Rifkind JM. Hemorheological changes during human aging. Gerontology 1998; 44:111-20.

55. Simpson LO, O'Neill DJ. Red cell shape changes in the blood of people 60 years of age and older, imply a role for blood rheology in the aging process. Gerontology 2003; 49:310-5.

56. Ellis NR, Nasser S, Wrighton RJ. A survey of the use of vitamin B12 in general practice. The Practitioner 1970; 204:838-42.

57. Ellis NR, Nasser S. A pilot study of vitamin B12 in the treatment of tiredness. Br J Nutr 1973; 30:277-83.

58. Jason LA, Torres-Harding SR, Jurgens A, et al. Comparing the Fukuda et al. criteria and the Canadian case definition for chronic fatigue syndrome. J Chr Fat Synd 2004; 12:37-52.

59. Myhill S, Booth NE, McLaren -Howard J. Chronic fatigue syndrome and mitochondrial dysfunction. Int J Clin Exp Med 2009; 2: 1-16.

CHAPTER V - RAMSAY'S DISEASE (ME): WHY AND HOW PEOPLE BECOME UNWELL

Introduction

Because our work has shown changes in the flow properties of blood samples from ME people (and also in other chronic disorders) it is important for sufferers to understand the implications of such changes and their significance in ill health.

In his 1892 textbook of physiology, (1) the father of British physiology, Professor Earnest Starling stated, "The capillaries may be regarded as the chief part of the circulation since the whole object of the varied arrangements of the heart and arterioles is to secure an adequate flow of blood through these smaller vessels – that is a supply of blood adequate to meet the needs of tissues in which the capillaries are embedded."

Although much information about the nature of capillaries has accumulated since 1892, there is little general recognition that changes in the blood itself also determine the rate of capillary blood flow which in turn determines whether or not there, "...*is a supply of blood adequate to meet the needs of tissues in which the capillaries are embedded.*" Thus, to a major degree, the metabolic needs of tissues are reflected in the simplicity or complexity of their capillary system. This was well illustrated in a Japanese study of the microvasculature of an important part of the brain (the hypothalamus) which revealed an incredibly complex microcirculation.(2) This complex capillary system is consistent with the fact that the brain and nerves are very sensitive to the oxygen deprivation which would follow any reduction in the rate of blood flow in the brain.

Resting muscles have a relatively low need for oxygen and nutrient substrates, but when stimulated to work, extra oxygen and substrates are needed to provide the energy needed for the muscle to perform its task. A reduction in the rate of capillary blood flow may so reduce the rate of oxygen delivery as to stimulate a switch from aerobic respiration to anaerobic respiration, with a reduced energy output and the production of lactic acid which may be accompanied by pain.

Because of the important role they play in determining whole body function, the secreting glands of the endocrine system are dependent upon normal rates of capillary blood flow to sustain the production of their secretions. **Therefore, if the rate of capillary blood flow fails to meet the metabolic needs of secreting glands, then body-wide dysfunction may follow.**

In ME people, when the flow properties of blood are abnormal (except during remissions when the blood returns to normal) it is not surprising that most report dysfunction of the central nervous system, muscles and overall weariness.

In terms of blood flow, the most important feature of capillaries is the internal diameter, and depending upon the technique used it has been claimed that the average diameter of a capillary lies between three and five microns. The significance of this value is that it is about one half of the diameter of a red blood cell, which means that in order to traverse a capillary bed, red cells must be able to change shape (to deform) so that they can squeeze through capillaries. It is possible that this is an important feature in the delivery of oxygen. In normal situations, red cell deformation occurs with an intra-capillary pressure of about 15 mm mercury. The extent to which red cells could deform without rupturing was reported in a paper with the intriguing title, "The spurting of erythrocytes through junctions of the vascular endothelium treated with Habu snake venom." (3) Transmission electron microscopy was used to illustrate the consequences of the intense vaso-constriction induced by habu snake venom, and showed that the dramatic increase in intra-capillary pressure had forced red cells through capillary walls. Although the cells were almost thread-like in form, they had not ruptured.

Because most capillaries will be smaller than the diameter of red cells, and as demonstrated, red cells can be extremely deformable, such observations draw attention to the importance of red cell deformability. Much has been written on this topic and PubMed listed 2133 papers written on the topic since 1969, which includes descriptions of techniques used to assess red cell deformability. However, there are many conflicting reports from studies using a variety of techniques, but in most cases the conflicting observations are explicable in terms of the pre-treatments of red cells prior to assessment. We and many others found the simple technique of Reid et al (4) provided reproducible results, provided that the anti-coagulated blood samples were filtered within an hour of the sample being drawn.

Because red cells lose the nucleus as they leave the bone marrow, they are incapable of independent existence and they respond to change in their environment by changing shape. Miller et al (5) reported that they were unable to prevent red cells from changing shape, even in their own plasma in a refrigerator. A high school girl showed that after five minutes in normal saline, her cells with altered margins (echinocytes) had been nearly eliminated and there was a marked increase in biconcave discocytes.(6) For that reason it is not surprising that techniques which assess the deformability of saline-washed red cells show high levels of deformability.

Such observations imply that three factors determine the rate of capillary blood flow: firstly, the internal diameter of the capillary; secondly, the deformability of red blood cells; thirdly, the intra-capillary pressure. Of these factors, only red cell deformability is relatively amenable to treatment. In 1974, Kury et al (7) used a spin-labelling technique to show that prostaglandin E1 improved red cell membrane fluidity. Evening primrose oil contains gammalinolenic acid, a precursor to prostaglandin E1, and in a study of atopy, Manku et al (8) reported that a minimum of four grams daily of evening primrose oil was needed to produce a significant increase in the blood levels of prostaglandin E1. Rasmussen et al, reported that while prostaglandin E1 improved blood filterability, the inflammatory prostaglandin E2 made red cells poorly filterable.(9) For these reasons, people with chronic ME may benefit from four grams daily of evening primrose oil.

Several studies have drawn attention to the beneficial effects on red cell flexibility, of fish oil containing high proportions of eicosapentaenoic acid. Having shown previously, by means of a spin-labelling technique, that the membranes of diabetic red cells were stiff and viscous, Kamada et al (10) reported that dietary supplementation with sardine oil so improved the fluidity of diabetic red cells that those cells could not be distinguished from the cells of non-diabetics. Although a three-month long trial of 4 grams of fish oil daily produced several benefits for subjects 65 years of age and older, some of the observed benefits did not persist, and for that reason at least 6 grams of fish oil daily is recommended. There are published studies in which 10 grams daily were used and another study concluded that the maximal tolerable daily dose was 21 grams daily. At the present time, fish oil and omega-3 fatty acids are "fashionable" although there is no recognition of their potential to improve blood flow by increasing the deformability of red blood cells.

A prescription drug, TRENTAL (pentoxifylline) has been shown to lower blood viscosity and to increase red cell deformability. For example, it was found that after taking 1200mg of TRENTAL daily for fourteen days, the red cell deformability of ten maturity-onset diabetics was increased significantly, without change in the phosphatide levels of the red cell membranes. (11) In a four-year-long study of diabetics treated with TRENTAL, the beneficial effects of improving capillary blood flow were marked by the fact that not a single complication of the diabetic state developed in four years. (12)

It is a great pity that there are no controlled studies of any of these agents in the treatment of ME, although Behan et al (13) reported beneficial effects of evening primrose oil containing a small amount of fish oil, in patients with post-viral fatigue. Possibly because of the lack of interest or of opportunity to carry out placebo-controlled trials of these three agents in ME people, it is not possible to identify with certainty which patients will respond to what treatment. Therefore, whatever treatment is chosen, it is necessary to assess the situation after six weeks of treatment. Unless there is a clearly perceived benefit, that treatment should be stopped and another agent tried.

The possible importance of observations which show that improving red cell deformability increases the rate of capillary blood flow and improves patient well-being, is that such observations draw attention to the capillary systems involved. After finding high proportions of cells with altered margins (echinocytes) in blood samples from two healthy, asymptomatic men, which implied that they had larger-than usual capillaries, it was proposed that

> ...subjects with the symptom of tiredness and high percentages of nondiscocytic cells in their blood would have smaller-than-usual capillaries, i.e. those with mean capillary diameters falling in the first quartile of a size distribution. Subjects with this characteristic would always be at risk of red-cell-shape-related impairment of capillary blood flow. Because of the difficulties of assessing capillary dimension, it

is emphasised that the data from red cell shape analysis should not be used in a predictive fashion (14).

However, since that was written, it has been found that when altered shape populations of red cells can be demonstrated, SPECT scans show reductions in regional cerebral blood flow.

What has this to do with ME?

It is proposed that people who develop ME have the anatomical feature of smaller-than-usual capillaries in those parts of the body which become dysfunctional and manifest symptoms, after exposure to an agent which initiates changes in the shape populations of red blood cells. Such a proposal provides a basis for understanding the near-random distribution of symptoms as well as emphasising that the term 'cure' is irrelevant. Even after an apparent recovery, people with small capillaries remain at risk. In addition, some other factor is involved. That factor is responsible for the long-term changes in the shape changes of red cells, but is able to 'switch off' and allow remissions which may be brief or long-lasting, before being 'switched on.' At this time, nothing is known about the identity of the factor (s) although it has been found that during remissions, the shape populations of red cells return to normal, implying that there is a normalising of the internal environment. Relapses are accompanied by a return to abnormal shape populations of red cells. As there are several other chronic disorders with changed shape populations of red cells, it is possible that they are separable on their symptoms.

Ramsay was impressed by the nature of the muscle dysfunction, the memory problems and the states of confusion which might reflect reduced blood flow in some cerebral region. He also recognised circulatory impairment as an ME problem. The suggestion that the central nervous system problems of ME sufferers are due to reduced blood flow in some region of the brain, is compatible with those SPECT observations which showed that different psychiatric disorders had different regions in the brain with reduced rates of cerebral blood flow.

While it is possible that the presence of small capillaries can account for the majority of ME cases, such a situation is unlikely to explain why prominent sports people have been stricken with ME. Unfortunately I have never had a blood sample for red cell shape analysis from any such cases. Because such cases are usually very unwell and greatly dysfunctional, it is possible that they are manifesting the effects of two possible changes. Firstly, that they had suffered a very dramatic response to an agent which stimulated a very high degree of change in red cell shape, so that the rate of blood flow, even in large capillaries was impaired. Secondly, that the nature of the red cell shape change was associated with reduced rates of uptake and delivery of oxygen. The combined effects of such changes could produce similar levels of dysfunction to those whose primary problem was small capillaries. However, it is possible that sports people with ME would undergo a complete recovery, although I have never seen any reports of long-term follow-up of such cases.

Although the small number of blood samples from children that I have assessed showed changed-shape populations of red cells, the smallness of the sample makes it unwise to comment on their relevance. In terms of the outcome, it seems that those who had ME in their teens or early twenties were most likely to have recovered sufficiently to be working full-time and be symptom free. Individuals who were in their mid-twenties to early forties when they were diagnosed have greatly varied outcomes. Some women were living a relatively normal lifestyle, albeit secluded, while at the other extreme some cases were bed-bound or house-bound. Less than twenty percent of this age group were working full time. The most seriously disadvantaged group had been diagnosed when they were more than fifty years of age. Possibly this reflects the combined effects of the ME-related and the age-related changes in the flow properties of blood, but about five percent of cases were in full time employment.

How does ME relate to other chronic disorders?

The changed red cell shape populations observed in blood samples from people with ME are not unique, as similar changes were reported in muscular dystrophy and in Huntington's Disease in the 1970s, followed by a study of spinocerebellar degeneration in 1983. None of those reports stimulated a study of the effects of such cells on blood flow. In fact, a 1985 report concerning cognition and cerebral blood flow in Huntington's Disease did not refer to the earlier study showing changed shape populations of red cells. Red cell shape analysis has revealed changed shape populations in a wide range of chronic states such as aging, AIDS, arachnoiditis, arthritis, attention deficit and hyper-reactivity disorder, bipolar disorder, cancer, CFS, diabetes (both types 1 and 2), Down syndrome, multiple sclerosis and repetitive strain disorder. It seems reasonable to conclude that until the problems of blood flow are addressed in individuals suffering from those disorders, their quality of life will be less than the best.

Conclusion

The objective of this book is to separate those with Ramsay's Disease (ME) from other disorders with changed red cell shape populations, in terms of Ramsay's criteria of muscle and central nervous system dysfunction with circulatory impairment. Such an objective should be achievable, as it was possible to diagnose ME prior to the introduction of CFS, and reductions in regional cerebral blood flow can be demonstrated by SPECT scans. There is abundant information to challenge the claims that ME is "…all in the head" and that it can be treated by behavioural modification and exercise. **Until those challenges are mounted successfully, the health problems of ME people will continue to be managed inappropriately.**

Chapter V References

1. Starling E. Elements of human physiology. J & A Churchill, London, 1892, p196.
2. Murikami T, Kikuta A, Iguchi T, et al. Blood vascular architecture of the rat cerebral hypophysis and hypothalamus. A dissection and scanning electron microscopy of vascular casts. Arch Histol Jap 1987; 50:133-76.
3. Ohsaka A, Suzuki K, Ohashi M. The spurting of erythrocytes through junctions of the vascular endothelium treated with habu snake venom. Microvasc Res 1975; 10:208-18.
4. Reid HL, Barnes AJ, Lock PJ, et al. A simple method for measuring erythrocyte deformability. J Clin Path 1976; 29:855-8.
5. Miller SE, Roses AD, Appel SH. Scanning electron microscope studies in muscular dystrophy. Arch Neurol 1976; 33:172-4.
6. Simpson LO. Red cell shape. NZ Med J 1993; 106:531. (Letter)
7. Kury PG, Ramwell PW, McConnell HM. The effects of prostaglandins E1 and E2 on the human erythrocyte as monitored by spin labels. Biochim Biophys Res Commun 1974; 56:478-83.
8. Manku MS, Horrobin D, Morse N, et al. Reduced levels of prostaglandin precursors in the blood of atopic patients: defective delta-6-desaturase function as a biochemical basis for atopy. Prost Leuko Med 1982; 9: 615-28
9. Rasmussen H, Lake W, Allen JE. The effects of catecholamines and prostaglandins upon human and rat erythrocytes. Biochim Biophys Acta 1975; 411:63-73.
10. Kamada T, Yamashita T, Baba Y, et al. Dietary sardine oil increases erythrocyte fluidity in diabetic patients. Diabetes 1986, 35:604-11.
11. Schubotz R, Muhlfelner O. The effect of pentoxifylline on erythrocyte deformability and on phosphatide fatty acid distribution in the erythrocyte membrane. Curr Med Res Opin 1977; 4: 609-17.
12. Ferrari E, Fioravanti M, Patti AL, et al. Effects of long-term treatment (4 years) with pentoxifylline on haemorheological changes and vascular complications in diabetic patients. Pharmatherapeutica 1987; 5:26-39.
13. Behan PO, Behan WMH, Horrobin D. Effects of high doses of essential fatty acids on the post-viral fatigue syndrome.
14. Simpson LO. Chronic tiredness and idiopathic chronic fatigue – a connection? NJ Med 1992; 89:211-6.

BACKGROUND TO THE CONTROVERSIES
SOME IMPORTANT CONCEPTS

In this section of the book, I attempt to provide an explanation of the concepts needed to understand and evaluate the medical and political controversies which surround this illness, and why you may find yourself treated in ways which may be either helpful or unhelpful. In the UK people who have ME could be considered particularly unfortunate because of the influence which the psychiatric lobby has been permitted to exercise within the Medical Research Council, in the NHS, and in the Department of Work and Pensions, and also because of its undue influence on the media. [9] [20]

However, you may come across individual G.P.s, nurses, cognitive behaviour therapists, occupational therapists and physiotherapists who understand your illness, and, in carrying out their functions, display respect for you and a spirit of collaboration with your own efforts to manage your illness and–work towards recovery. If at all possible, seek out such helpers.

As well as providing you with a vocabulary of concepts and terms, this section will include recommendations, for doctors, psychotherapists, and public policy

In a few minor respects my thinking or use of terminology may differ from Dr. Simpson's. We both agree that the classification 'Chronic Fatigue Syndrome' is a rag-bag collection of unrelated medical or psychiatric problems, whereas 'Myalgic Encephalomyelitis' – ME, or Ramsay's Disease – is a very specific, clearly distinguishable, physiologically-based illness. In using the term 'Chronic Fatigue Syndrome', some authors intend it to include ME, while some define it in such a way that ME can actually be excluded. For example, in the Oxford Criteria, 'post-exertional fatigue', generally regarded as a defining feature of ME, is listed as one of a number of symptoms which may be present, but its presence is not required for the patient to be diagnosed as having CFS. So many people given that diagnostic label may not have ME. And it is rumoured that the (unpublished) 'London' criteria, used for selection of patients in the PACE Trial, may have excluded patients who experienced 'post exertional fatigue'. If this were the case, none of the subjects of that study had ME!

Where Dr. Simpson and I differ is in our emphasis: Dr. Simpson would generally take the view that any reference to CFS suggests the author is dealing with conditions that exclude ME; while if what is being researched sounds to me like a description of ME, but the author is calling it CFS (or CFS/ME, or ME/CFS), I am more likely to give the benefit of the doubt and assume that what is being discussed is ME.

Classification

Classification is necessary in order for us to make sense of our world. Here is a black telephone. I could classify it among objects which are black, along with the mouse, the keyboard, my glasses case, my piano, and my trousers. Or I could classify it as a means of communication, along with my mobile phone and my PC. Neither form of classification is 'wrong', but the first will be more useful if I am planning a colour scheme, the second if I am making plans to do with communication.

The classification of plants and animals began with identifying things in terms of their superficial similarities and differences. Things with similar shapes and similar structures were placed in the same class. Developments in science and technology have provided us with far more sophisticated methods of classification – DNA-based classification has thrown up many surprises and revealed many apparently improbable connections. We need to be aware that **external similarities do not necessarily indicate that things belong in the same category.**

Medical Classification

The same principle applies to medical classification. A particular symptom (for example, a headache) can occur in a range of conditions, some of them relatively trivial and some life-threatening. Although the presentation of symptoms is the same, the underlying causes may be widely different.

Further, we now understand that many illnesses are caused by bacteria, and others are caused by viruses. Although the symptoms may be similar, antibiotic treatment will be effective for bacterial infections, but it will not be helpful if the illness is caused by a virus. Now that we are aware of the problems caused by antibiotic overuse, doctors are encouraged to respect this distinction, and to help patients to understand that antibiotic treatment is not relevant to viral illnesses, for example, common colds, or flu. Classification by the cause of an illness (the aetiopathology) offers the possibility of more accurate and effective treatment.

Diagnosis

Because any specific symptom may occur in a variety of illnesses, diagnosis requires further information. One source of further information is the pattern, or **constellation of symptoms** which indicates a particular condition. A headache on its own may be a consequence of temporary stress, or, along with a stuffy nose and a cough, it may be indicative of a common cold. A headache accompanied by a high fever and a particular kind of rash could indicate meningitis, which will require immediate treatment. Another constellation of symptoms that we have been encouraged to recognise in a recent UK TV campaign is encapsulated in the acronym FAST – face drooping on one side, a limp arm, speech difficulty, time to ring the emergency services – this is likely to be a stroke.

Another way of arriving at an accurate diagnosis is to consider the **history** of the individual experiencing it. If a person has a history of mild headaches associated with particular stressful events, then another headache associated with a stressful event is likely to be more of the same. However, a headache occurring in the absence of a stressful event, in a different part of the head, of different intensity, accompanied by other symptoms previously absent would warrant further investigation. A good diagnostician, like a good detective, pays close attention to the details, and avoids jumping to conclusions. Any **departure from a usual pattern,** either the appearance of symptoms in a normally healthy individual, or a new symptom or set of symptoms in a person who already has health problems, **warrants careful investigation.**

Diagnosis by List

A growing emphasis is being placed on the importance of statistical analysis. This means that research has to be designed to produce quantifiable, countable units of data. Diagnosis can then consist of taking the statistical results of researches concerning a particular condition and turning them into a checklist of symptoms. These may then become protocols for diagnosis which leave no room for the diagnostician's human judgement. They cannot take account of variable and complex circumstances in individual cases, or consider the history or narrative of an illness. This is particularly the case in psychiatry, which I discuss further below.

It will be evident, as well, that patients encountering this narrow, statistically and technologically-based approach in their doctors will be tempted to turn to practitioners who will take a more holistic approach to their situations.

Treatment or Symptom-Relief?

We commonly 'treat' headaches with over-the-counter painkillers, colds with decongestants and paracetamol and mild allergies with antihistamines. These remedies address the symptoms – pain, stuffy nose, itchy eyes or skin. They do not address the causes of the headache, cold or allergy.

It is important to distinguish this, **symptom-relief**, from the kind of **treatment** which is intended to 'cure' an illness – for example, antibiotics to kill the bacteria which are the cause of infections, or antiviral medication for conditions caused by a virus.

For life-threatening illnesses, such as meningitis or pneumonia, the **use of symptom-relief can endanger the patient** by temporarily disguising the symptoms while the underlying cause is continuing to operate.

That is why a good doctor will not prescribe until she or he is satisfied that a correct diagnosis has been made. To use an extreme example, if a person has a headache which is caused by a developing brain tumour, the use of pain relief may delay a diagnosis until it is too late to treat the tumour successfully. The same thing can happen with a symptom such as a cough, or stomach-ache. This is why most over-the-counter medications will have a warning that if the symptom continues over a certain length of time, you must stop taking it and see your G.P.

Treatment or Rehabilitation?

We've mentioned the constellation of symptoms which indicate the possibility of a stroke.

A stroke needs immediate treatment directed at dealing with the blood clot or haemorrhage which is causing the symptoms. **Once that cause has been dealt with, it will become appropriate to instigate a programme of rehabilitation,** designed to help the patient regain as much use of muscles and speech as possible, in an attempt to overcome the damage which has been caused by the stroke. Clearly it would not be advisable to confuse the two, and try a programme of rehabilitation before the cause of the problem has been resolved – in fact it could be quite dangerous.

A broken limb or torn muscle would also be a situation in which some degree of healing would have to have taken place before it would be advisable or safe to begin a programme of rehabilitation.

And note that the techniques used for rehabilitation of muscles (of which Graded Exercise Therapy is one) work on the assumption that the aerobic muscle metabolism is functioning normally. Forcing exercise on muscles which are using the anaerobic metabolic system will create damage, not repair.

Psychiatric Diagnosis

As a psychotherapist, I consider skill at psychiatric diagnosis to be essential. It is not true that because we only deal with emotional issues, a faulty diagnosis cannot endanger the physical health or even the lives of patients. If we do not make a careful distinction between symptoms which have a cause that we can discover within the circumstances of the patient's life, and symptoms which may have a physical cause, we may fail to refer our patient for a needed medical investigation. In such a case, a psychotherapist or psychiatrist might offer the kind of symptom relief that proves fatal because a physical problem has not been diagnosed and treated. Epilepsy, multiple sclerosis, duodenal ulcers are among the illnesses wrongly labelled as psychiatric in the past, and patients still lose their lives because, for example, symptoms of a brain tumour are mistakenly diagnosed.

Unfortunately, the diagnostic manuals which are commonly used in psychiatry, most notably, the American Diagnostic and Statistical Manual (DSM) are completely dominated by the tick-list approach to diagnosis. (A discussion about this can be found in the booklet 'Articles on Diagnostic and Statistical Manual of Mental Disorders, Including: Structured Clinical Interview for DSM-IV, DSM-5', produced by Hephaestus Books [20]) This approach has apparently replaced clinical judgements based on a thorough, sensitive, and in-depth interview with the patient, including careful attention to the history and narrative of the illness, both from childhood onward and in terms of the patient's current circumstances. In the past few years, the psychiatric lobby has created a new list, to be included under the DSM category 'Somatoform Disorders' with the intention of getting what they call CFS/ME included in this category as a psychiatric condition. If their enterprise is successful, and it may already have been successful, this new categorisation will be included in the next edition, DSM-5, which is due to come out in 2013. [21] [22]

The ongoing attempt to classify ME as a psychiatric condition neglects the fact that a psychiatric diagnosis must include an explanatory history. The narrative of most mental illness is a history of negative environmental factors and events dating from childhood and/or highly stressful or traumatic contemporary events. Compare this with the narrative of people with ME, which in many cases is that of an energetic, hard-working, ambitious individual who is generally successful in life activities and has always ignored or risen above physical complaints. This is not the narrative of a depressed or anxious person, or of a hypochondriac, or of a person who would prefer 'a career' as an invalid. For such an individual to be, relatively suddenly, and for no evident reason, rendered extremely disabled, is a clear indication that some form of serious physical illness is involved. Of course, in their determination to keep people with ME in their own hands, the psychiatric lobby have now defined being conscientious and hard-working as a predisposing factor, along with being a woman. For a detailed discussion of these factors, see [23] (A recent look at the DSM 5 website reveals that they have now declared that a person can be given a diagnosis of 'somatoform disorder' even if a) they do have a medical condition and b) don't have any history of trauma. This is based on the a priori assumption that CFS is a somatoform disorder. [22]. But this is contested by Dr. Allen Frances, see 'DSM In Distress – Mislabelling Medical Illness Mental Disorder'. [24]

Ramsay's Disease: Back to Classification

In the accounts which Dr. Simpson gives of various attempts to create diagnostic lists for what was renamed 'Chronic Fatigue Syndrome' two things are evident.

Firstly, the lists do not convey any sense of coherence in terms of a physiological understanding of CFS/ME, or any sense of coherence in terms of a claim that CFS/ME is a psychiatric problem. They are just lists. The other evident feature is that the lists are broad enough in scope to include a range of conditions which are not ME, and to include psychiatric conditions, particularly depression. (Questionnaires purporting to diagnose depression which include physical symptoms of CFS/ME not related to mood help to further muddy the waters. [25])

The Effect of These Classifications on Research

With such a broad and incoherent collection of symptoms included under the term 'CFS/ME' and its variants, it is highly likely that any research based on studying groups of people who have been chosen according to this categorisation may be largely, or completely irrelevant to people who have ME. It is notable that the Oxford criteria include, but do not require, the symptom 'post exertion malaise', which in most writing about ME is considered a defining feature. This omission means that if a research cohort is chosen on the basis of the Oxford criteria (and I believe that the recent PACE trial, discussed in detail below, is an example), it will necessarily include people who have other conditions, and may even exclude anyone suffering from ME. When it is reported that studies have a high drop-out rate, it seems even more likely that people who have ME and have therefore found themselves unable to continue with the trial might not have their numbers included in the final report. (Defenders of the PACE Trial insist this has not happened.) This could serve to explain the production of statistics purporting to show that graded exercise therapy (GET) is helpful, not harmful, for people with ME.

(As of February, 2013, Queen Mary College is appealing against a Freedom of Information ruling that they must release information about deterioration found in subjects of the PACE Trial. [26])

A parallel scenario might be a drugs trial in which patients who experienced side-effects and therefore dropped out of the research programme were not included in the final statistics. The authors could then report 'research has shown' that side-effects are rare.

These distortions, which can render research valueless, are one of the main reasons why Dr. Simpson is of the firm belief that we should revert to Ramsay's original criteria for diagnosis, and that the illness should be renamed 'Ramsay's Disease (ME)'.

LESLIE O. SIMPSON & NANCY BLAKE

Ramsay's Disease: Diagnosis

The constellation of symptoms presented by people who have Ramsay's Disease (ME) can easily be confused with a random list of symptoms presented by a person who worries about every little thing and is constantly bothering their doctor for diagnostic tests. The assumption of those who would consign us to a psychiatric category now called 'somatoform symptom disorder' is that that person is who we are.

The main feature of this constellation is problems with muscle function that seem to indicate that the aerobic metabolism is not functioning properly. This malfunction means that the muscles are deprived of oxygen, so that the body has recourse to the anaerobic muscle metabolism (usually reserved for extremely demanding physical tasks, and accompanied by a build-up of lactic acid) in order to perform even the most minimal physical exertion. The delayed and disabling fatigue following such exertion is typical of the fatigue experienced by people who have performed extreme physical tasks, such as weight lifting, running marathons or mountain climbing. Another feature of the constellation is cognitive difficulties, sometimes described as 'brain fog', which is also indicative of oxygen deprivation in the cognitive areas in the brain. A third feature is dysregulation of body temperature, sleep rhythms, and appetite, indicating problems in the endocrine system, which also can most easily be explained by oxygen deprivation. A fourth feature is a set of symptoms (sore throat, swollen glands) indicative of immune system activation. A fifth feature is the variability of the symptoms, in which remissions occur, but the patient appears to remain vulnerable to re-activation of symptoms if over-exertion takes place.

Note that some elements in this description depart from Dr. Simpson's, although we are in fundamental agreement. I am ascribing the delayed and prolonged fatigue, which is the defining factor in ME, to oxygen deprivation and failure of removal of waste products having caused the anaerobic muscle metabolism to be activated, with the implication that minimal exertion, for a person with ME, equates to an extreme level of exertion in a normal person. This hypothesis seems to me to fit with Ramsay's first descriptive statement concerning ME: **A unique form of muscle fatigability whereby, even after a minor degree of physical effort, three, four or five days or longer elapse before full muscle power is restored.** I am adding endocrine dysregulation and symptoms of immune-system activation to the symptoms mentioned by Ramsay, although he did state at one stage that he thought that the immune system was implicated.

Historically, this very complex but consistent constellation has appeared in disparate and sometimes quite isolated geographical areas, in people, including children, who have no prior knowledge of ME. It would be interesting to get a statistician's (or a bookie's!) view on the odds that anything this complicated could be conjured up just because the individuals involved had suddenly decided that being disabled and in pain would be more rewarding than leading their previously happy and successful lives, as is claimed by the Wessely School. [7]

It is also very puzzling that the medical community, many of whom have been personally informed about Dr. Simpson's extensive and carefully conducted research continue to fail to acknowledge its existence.

Ramsay's Disease: Back to Symptoms Versus Causes

Dr. Simpson's work on blood viscosity explains most of the symptoms of ME. His observations also show that when symptoms of ME are in remission, the red blood cell population returns to a normal proportion of biconcave discocytes. His work does not purport to explain the underlying causes of this illness. However, trying the treatments he suggests will alleviate symptoms in a percentage of people who have ME because they address the <u>cause of the symptoms</u>, although <u>not the underlying cause of the illness itself</u>, which remains unknown.

Ramsay's Disease: Treatment Versus Symptom Relief

Dr. Simpson's suggestions lie somewhere between treatment and symptom relief. They are not simply symptom relief in the sense that taking a pain-killer for a headache would be. They address a physiological process, the changing shape of the red blood cells, which causes most of the symptoms. Following his recommendations offers a very good chance of improving an ME patient's ability to perform physical and cognitive tasks, in many cases effecting major improvements. But a treatment which would actually cure the illness remains to be discovered. The need for continuing research into physiological causes, conducted on a sample of people whose illness has been clearly defined as ME, is self-evident.

Ramsay's Disease: Treatment Versus Rehabilitation

As the causes of ME remain unknown, but are not psychiatric, there is no specific treatment which can address those causes, and we are still in the situation which Ramsay describes: a situation in which, after adopting Dr. Simpson's recommendations, rest, especially in the early stages, is the principal recommendation that we can make.

Actually, the word 'rest' sounds so much like a kind of passive 'giving up' that I much prefer to write about 'conservation of energy'. Given a sudden major loss of the ability to perform physical or cognitive acts, we need to retreat behind the barricades and actively plan how to conduct our lives with this very limited budget of usable energy. We need to appreciate first of all that whatever is attacking our system, our body needs all its resources to deal with it, and we need to think of 'resting' as an active strategy (see 'The Power of Rest', by Dr. M. Edlund [27]) for dealing with this illness: a good general's strategic retreat to allow his troops to regroup and recover – surrendering the battle in order to win the war. **Fighting against this illness in the way that medicine and convention expect us to will ensure that we lose not only the battle but also the war – in the short term, we will get worse. In the long term, we may end up among the 25% who are completely disabled.**

Cognitive Behaviour Therapy, if practiced as recommended by the psychiatric lobby, encourages patients to ignore their symptoms, and to relinquish their 'belief' that their illness is physical and that exercise will harm them. It is evident that if practised in this way, psychological treatment will be encouraging the patient in some false beliefs which, if acted on, will certainly make them worse.

Graded Exercise Therapy is based on the same set of false beliefs, with the added false belief that the muscles of a person who has ME will respond to exercise in the way that the muscles of a healthy individual would respond – by building strength. This is even more damaging – trying to force muscles to work in the absence of oxygen and with a build-up of waste products will simply cause harm.

Graded Exercise may be an appropriate recommendation for the rehabilitation of people whose muscles have been damaged, and are healing, or have healed, **as long as the aerobic metabolic system is functioning normally. This is not the case in ME, and therefore Graded Exercise is not just inappropriate, but harmful.** [16] [28]

If Cognitive Behaviour Therapy was intended to assist the person with ME to work within the limits of the illness without losing self-respect, and become very creative about how to manage life with ME, it could be helpful.

In my case, I was also able to make use of a technique from neurolinguistic psychotherapy called 're-framing'. My father, a classic Type A energetic, overdriven personality, died suddenly of a coronary heart attack at the age of sixty-two. I am like my father both physically and psychologically and I may have been similarly at risk of an early death. My thoughts were that 'if I have to lie down for five years, at least I'm not going to die of a heart attack'. This enabled me to 'frame' ME as a form of protection. Of course the 'ME is all in your head' brigade could spring on this thought as evidence that my way of thinking was encouraging the illness, when in fact, it was one way not to go mad from the frustration and boredom which ME imposed.

If we accept that ME is a long illness, and that it has a relapsing/remitting course, the question of appropriate rehabilitation becomes very complex indeed. Often we (people who have ME) cheerfully embark on some project intended to improve our well-being and build up our stamina, experience some benefits, feel delighted, carry on doing the same things, and find ourselves becoming ill again. Very careful attention to limits can mean a gradual progress towards becoming more well, but this progress is likely to have marked ups and downs. We are in more danger of harming ourselves through ill-advised attempts at rehabilitation than we are if we resist such programmes, at least until we have learned from our experience of the relapses which too much enthusiasm can cause. Dr. Acheson's statement is unequivocal: **"The association of premature rehabilitation with relapse is well described."** [29]

Ramsay's Disease: Research

We have covered a good deal of medical terminology and concepts concerning ME. Now I would like to turn to the issues concerning research.

Today, many people in the UK who are educated, well-informed, and concerned about contemporary issues will have the impression that the 'scientific' view of ME is that it is not a physiological entity, but entirely a psychological construct. Their impression will be that the idea that ME is a physiologically-based illness which belongs in the area of unproven, unscientific, alternative or complementary medical thinking. In their terms, they will 'know' that 'scientists' have now 'proved scientifically' that it is psychological.

Of course, this will only be the case if they have not themselves experienced ME, or been close to someone who has. Personal experience of this illness revises such beliefs radically and immediately – as would, of course, a careful review of all the biomedical research that has been done, including an assessment of the weakness of the evidence that any psychiatric component is involved. See Komaroff's Review [17] of Manu's book on functional psychiatric disorders, in which it appears that Manu began his review believing that ME was psychiatric, and, after studying the literature, concluded that it was not.

If we ask how this climate of opinion has come about, one answer is that the group of psychiatrists who have gained influence with the government and with major insurers have done everything they can to create it. (A detailed account of this process is given in the document Corporate Collusion? by Professor Malcolm Hooper et al. [9]) This article includes discussion of the limitations imposed on the authors of the York Review of literature on CFS/ME. This review, under the leadership narrowly focused on reports of the type of trials used by the psychiatrists, ignoring thousands of biomedical research papers, is usually cited by government officials in response to queries about the status of this illness within the NHS.)

To understand how the psychiatric lobbyists have managed to achieve this outcome, we need to consider how biomedical research is conducted.

The most basic approach is to start with a hypothesis about cause and effect, and to set up an experiment to see whether intervention A does, in a carefully constructed, meticulously recorded situation, result in the observation of effect B, and how often this is the case (the statistical probability). You report this work, and perhaps other researchers follow your directions carefully, and record whether A results in B at roughly the same level of probability. If enough other researchers come to the same conclusions, then "A, following this procedure, will result in B, at x level of probability" becomes established as a 'scientific fact'. The robustness of this conclusion is enhanced by the requirement that research reported in reputable scientific journals is 'peer-reviewed', which means the submitted reports are sent to other researchers in the field for their critical opinions, which will influence whether or not the research is published.

However, a danger that is now recognised is the possibility of 'observer bias', where the researcher's own expectations or pre-conceptions can affect how the data are perceived and recorded, thereby influencing the outcome of the research, and steps need to be taken to detect and exclude this. As the systems studied become more complex, moving from physics through chemistry, biology, medicine, and the social sciences, the simple proposition "A plus the stated procedure will give B at this level of probability" becomes much more difficult to separate out from a multitude of possible influences, including observer bias.

The 'gold standard' for any research involving human subjects, especially into medical effects, is considered to be the 'random-controlled double-blind' experiment. At its simplest, some 'treatment' (usually a drug) will be given to half your subjects and a 'placebo', a physiologically inert substance, to the other half. An attempt will be made to match your group of subjects with the 'controls' (the ones getting the placebo) – same gender or age distribution, same illness at the same stage, etc. 'Random' here refers to a method (usually computer-generated) for choosing randomly which subjects get the treatment and which the placebo, and 'double-blind' refers to precautions taken to ensure that neither the subjects themselves nor the researchers giving out the pills know who gets which.

The final outcome is meant to give an unbiased as possible set of figures showing to what extent subjects were helped by the treatment compared with the placebo. However, even if the 'random-controlled double-blind' procedure is adhered to rigorously, what the results mean can depend crucially on whether the choice of matters to probe is appropriate

LESLIE O. SIMPSON & NANCY BLAKE

to the population being studied, and whether the researchers are aware of the choices they have made, and how these can affect the validity of their conclusions.

Psychiatrists, psychologists, and social scientists figure prominently among researchers who attempt to observe strict 'random-controlled double-blind' protocols, or at least 'random controlled trials, and these are referred to as 'the gold standard' for research. These areas of study are, however, particularly unsuited to this approach. How would either researchers or subjects be kept from knowing which were getting some form of treatment and which were simply left on a waiting list (a common way to form a 'control group')? Yet the term 'evidence-based' is often confined to studies which take this form.

Those who use methods such as Cognitive Behaviour Therapy have developed questionnaire scales for measuring improvement in their clients, and often use very complicated statistical procedures in analysing and reporting the results, which can make it difficult for the non-mathematically educated reader to evaluate the significance of the figures presented. In research based on the use of questionnaires, the design of these also has a measurable effect on the outcome of the investigation – questions examining the same issue can get very different responses, depending on how they are framed. Moreover, if the questioning is done in an interview setting, the subjects can often become aware of what answers the researcher would prefer to get, and this can also influence their replies. In some cases research may be based largely on self-reported information not verified by any objective physical measurement, and then it is especially open to both error and manipulation. [30]

On the biomedical side, there have, over the years, been several thousand research papers on ME, or ME/CFS, or CFS/ME, which have measured variations in a range of physiological factors. These have been done by virologists, immunologists, cardiologists, and geneticists, to name a few. (As ME is a multi-system illness, and medical training at an advanced level involves specialisation, each specialist will be conducting research within their own field, and this in itself probably places limits on our ability to gain an overall understanding of the illness.) The data obtained are generally compared with data on people who do not have the illness being studied, but in many (perhaps most) cases, these have not been strictly 'random-controlled double-blind' studies. The latter are sometimes referred to as 'evidence-based research', but this does not mean that all the other studies are not 'evidence-based' or that their results can or should be dismissed – if we do this, we are going to lose a great deal of pertinent and valid information. For one example of the number and quality of such research projects, see Margaret Williams' compilation of studies supporting 'The Immunological Basis of ME', in the Journal of the Invest in ME Conference of May, 2012 [31]

Clearly, however, if you do a review of the literature on ME in which you purposely exclude any research that is not a 'random controlled double blind' study, you will end up with many references to papers written by psychologists, psychiatrists and social scientists, but you will miss out much of the vast literature on laboratory studies that indicate physiological factors. According to the critique of the York Review referred to above, pressure was put on the researchers to confine their literature search in this way, thus facilitating the conclusion there is 'little evidence' that ME/CFS is a physiological illness.

And this is how we reach the paradoxical situation demonstrated, for example, in the CDC guidelines [32]: the list of symptoms of the illness includes becoming more ill after

200

physical or mental effort, yet this is followed by the 'evidence based' recommendation that the use of GET could be helpful. (As of 2012, this contrast has been made less evident.)

Citation Bias

Research scientists are aware that journal articles gain respect and credibility the more times they are cited by other authors. A recent article [10] has pointed out that if a substantial number of people supporting a particular theory publish papers in which each cites the work of the other (and they avoid any reference to published work which challenges their hypotheses), 'scientific credibility' for the theory can be created and strengthened even when no new research on it has actually been done. This effect is called 'citation bias'. (And, as in the example studied in the article referred to, this can happen even when the theory isn't, in fact, true in the first place.)

The research that has been done may even be flawed in various ways. An obvious flaw in testing treatment safety and efficacy is not to follow up individuals who drop out of trials. If they have dropped out because of side effects of the treatment, and they are not included in the final figures, this will clearly distort the statistics concerning the existence and seriousness of side-effects – and hence the 'safety' of the proposed treatment.

The Pace Trial

'Pacing, Activity, and Cognitive behavioural Evaluation' is the title of a study initiated by the UK Medical Research Council in 2003, which was strongly influenced (and partially subsidised) by proponents of the psychiatric model of ME. This trial has been a subject of ongoing controversy from the time it was first being proposed and funded and throughout the time it was being carried out. And it continues to be so, following its publication in The Lancet, in February of 2011. A detailed critique by Professor Malcolm Hooper in the form of a letter to the Lancet was published in part in a subsequent issue. The full document is also available on the ME Action website [33]. A number of other critiques also appeared in letters to Lancet: [34] [35] [36]

More recently, the Journal of Internal Medicine has published a review suggesting new international criteria for ME, giving a detailed account of much of the medical research that has been done, and strongly recommending that the neurological illness, ME, be taken out of the category CFS/ME in the NICE guidelines, because the treatments recommended there, CBT and GET, are inappropriate and potentially harmful for people with ME. [37]

For a very detailed critique of an article by Harvey and Wessely, which provides strong counterarguments to the position taken by those authors, see Maes and Twisk [19]. This article provides references to a number of other sources of support for the biomedical position, as well as to one explaining that, although major depression and ME have some common features, it is possible to differentiate the two with 100% accuracy. [38]

It may be coincidental that when a prestigious group of international researchers into ME have published guidelines that entirely support the physiological model of ME, and in response, there is much carefully thought-out criticism of the PACE Trial, Professor Wessely has been given a great deal of media attention for his complaints about receiving 'death threats', which he feels 'will inhibit research into ME.' (The PACE Trial was not research into ME, it was a very expensive exercise purporting to support the use of CBT and GET for people who have ME.) He further deplores the unwillingness of the ME community to accept that our illness is a psychiatric condition, because we are thus depriving ourselves of the possibility of 'completely reversing' our illness using his methods. He has thus diverted attention from the valid criticisms of the PACE Trial, and reinforced the public image of people who have ME as ungrateful hypochondriacs [39].

The PACE Trial can be criticised first of all for using the 'Oxford Criteria' in selecting the subject group. The Oxford Criteria do not require the delayed and protracted recovering time following exercise which was considered by Ramsay, and most researchers following him, as the definitive feature of ME. This means that there is no guarantee that the subjects studied actually had ME, rather than some other condition characterised by fatigue. (The criteria used were called the London criteria, and they have never been published, but it has been said that people suffering from post-exertional malaise were actually excluded from the PACE Trial – see Malcolm Hooper's letter to Lancet re the PACE Trial [33]])

A second criticism is that activity levels in the initial stages of the research were measured by the use of an actometer: a device which records actual movement. Subsequent measures of activity level were based on self-reported improvement only. There has been a research paper which has shown that self-reports of improvements in fatigue level have not been accompanied by increases in activity level, measured by actigraph [30]. It seems that by dropping the use of such a physical measure, self-reports of 'improvement' might leave the reader free to interpret 'improvement' as including improvement in levels of activity, when in fact such an interpretation is not justified. In any case, the improvements reported were slight, and in no way indicated that the illness had been 'completely reversed'. For example, the distance which the successfully treated (described as a return to 'normal') patients could walk in six minutes (379 metres) compares unfavourably with the distance (400 metres) which would qualify a person suffering from congestive lung disease to be put on a list for a lung transplant [33].

There have been accounts by PACE subjects in which they report pressure to give the answers the researchers clearly wanted them to give. These criticisms, and a much fuller discussion of the PACE Trial, can be found in Professor Hooper's response referred to above. Other detailed and well-founded criticisms were published in letters to Lancet following the initial publications of the PACE Results [34] [35] [36].

Recently Professor Wessely was the recipient of the John Maddox Award for courageously 'standing up for science'. Subsequent to this, Professor Wessely has received a knighthood for 'services to the mental health of veterans'. Apparently this includes insisting that Gulf War Syndrome is a psychiatric condition, and offering psychiatric services. Does this sound at all familiar? Many in the ME/CFS community are experiencing a combination of incredulity and despair. If you are at all puzzled by the ever-increasing power and influence of someone like Professor Wessely, there are a couple of references which I found enlightening. [40] [41]

Conclusion

I hope that the information and analysis offered in this chapter will have provided the reader with the concepts and references to further sources of information needed to make your own evaluations of what you read and hear about ME.

Suggestions for Managing the Doctor/Patient Relationship

The information provided in this book should be of considerable help to anyone who is either suffering from ME or anyone who is dealing with a patient who has ME. Our belief is that doctors and patients are on the same side in this endeavour, and this constructive relationship has in fact been shown to be helpful in itself in supporting the possibility of improvement. [23]

As a patient who has ME, you will first of all have to deal with the responses of your doctor. In my introduction, I referred to the two very different attitudes of the first doctors whom I consulted. The first was convinced that my symptoms were psychiatric, dismissed the information I presented, became angry about the article in the paper which explained ME, and concluded by saying that he would have to refer me to another doctor in the practice.

The second doctor, a woman, believed what I told her, apparently accepted that what I had was probably ME, gave me routine blood tests to exclude any other diagnosis, and told me simply to let her know when I needed a sick note in order to take time off from work. I did not become a problem to her, because I acknowledged that there was no direct diagnostic test for ME, and no treatment she could offer, so that self-management was the obvious option.

Dr. Dan Rutherford, in his account of ME on Netdoctor sets an admirable example of kindness, respect and consideration [42]

From a doctor's point of view, a patient who presents with the multiple and varying symptoms characteristic of ME, knows nothing about it, has no idea what is happening to them and is very upset about it is likely to be what has been described as 'the heart-sink' patient – the one the doctor dreads to see coming in the door! He/she will be demanding a clear diagnosis and an effective treatment (perfectly reasonable expectations, by the way!). Here is someone who is extremely disabled, often quite suddenly, with a controversial illness about which there is conflicting advice, but no definite tools to assist in diagnosis, and treatment recommendations towards which the patient is likely to be hostile. Not the easiest of situations!

Bearing in mind all the pressures on doctors, especially the limited time they have for each patient appointment, and the wider pressures on the NHS, perhaps you, the patient, will be able to sympathise with whatever response you may get from your doctor, even it may be not entirely helpful.

If your doctor simply rejects the whole concept of ME (doesn't 'believe it's a real illness') then clearly you need to be seeing someone else.

If your doctor follows the line recommended by NICE – that you should assure your patient that their symptoms are real – and then follow the rest of the NICE recommendations, including refusal of tests which would show the physiological manifestations of ME, and the recommendations for CBT and GET – you are in a difficult position.

If their attitude is generally sympathetic, and they genuinely wish to be helpful, it may be possible to establish a collaborative relationship in which they respect your account of your situation, and that you are doing what you believe to be best for your own recovery.

If, however, you are being pushed to do more than you can, or sent to a specialist service in which treatments are offered on a coercive basis, then you are in serious difficulties. Cooperating with such a regime is very likely to make you physically worse, while resisting it is likely to be interpreted as 'resistance' in the psychiatric sense – a determination to hold onto your illness. A classical double bind - with your future at stake – will you be allowed the 'space' to protect and preserve the possibility of long-term improvement, or will you be forced down a path to ultimate permanent disability?

You will need to develop high-order negotiating skills, or find someone who can exercise such skills on your behalf. My own good fortune is never to have been in such a situation, and my instinct is to follow the example of relatively defenceless creatures – adopt protective colouring, make yourself blend into the environment and become invisible, say a quiet and unassertive 'yes' to everything while doing, and not-doing whatever you sense is necessary for your self-preservation.

Whatever disability allowance you may have acquired is likely to be dependent on perceived cooperation. The irony of the way this illness is treated is that your genuine determination to recover as much as you can requires that you behave as though you are doing the opposite, ('just not trying') while appearing to cooperate with a regime which is likely to be making you worse. Quite a lot for a very sick person to manage!

Of course, if your doctor has had personal experience with ME, you will encounter a completely different level of understanding. He or she will know that your illness is genuine, and physical, and will understand how you need to manage your life. In that case, your doctor becomes an ally in helping you manage the necessary lifestyle changes and deal with the complexities of the wider system you are involved in – getting disability allowance while you need it, negotiating any necessary adaptations to enable you to return to work or to education.

In this case, you can reciprocate by respecting the limits on what even the most sympathetic doctor can offer, both in time and in terms of diagnostic procedures and treatment options. If you both accept that you have ME, then there is little more that your doctor can do for you.

The best possible outcome would be that your doctor can be persuaded to consider Dr. Simpson's information and recommendations. He or she might be interested in getting a micrograph of a sample of your blood to observe the red cell irregularities. Most importantly, you could be supported in a trial of Dr. Simpson's treatment recommendations, with the distinct possibility of an observable improvement in your well-being. One would hope that your doctor would be delighted to be able to offer something which will be demonstrably helpful.

Recommendations for Psychotherapists

As a psychotherapist, you will find that ME does not respond directly to any work which is based on the idea that the illness has its origins within the usual narratives of a psychological or psychiatric history, and this will confirm to you that the illness itself has its origins within dysfunctional physiological processes. The simple recognition of this fact can itself be helpful to your client – ME is difficult enough to figure out how to cope with, without also having to struggle against other people's 'false beliefs'!

Insofar as the NHS subscribes to the view that the illness can be 'safely and effectively' treated with CBT and GET, your client may be at risk of being made worse by the treatments which they are offered. The fact is that the prognosis for their long-term future depends on their minimising physical and mental exertion as much as possible during the early months of this very long-lasting illness. The importance of this cannot be over-emphasized: every bit of rest and every sacrifice of normal activity should be coded as a positive act which is contributing to the possibility of improving health in the longer term.

In recognition of this fact, your most important task is to assist your previously active, ambitious, energetic client in finding a way to cope with sudden and fairly extreme disability – paradoxically, by 'giving in'. This is very much against the grain of cultural expectations and is also likely to go against the grain of their own character. The challenge for the therapist is to help the person to 'give in' to the illness without losing self-respect or even losing a sense of 'who they are'.

Like most major health challenges, ME forces people to re-evaluate what is important, and what may have to be relinquished, within the context of their whole lives. Ways must be found to help them code elements of their new situation as offering opportunities to value new activities, and to feel valued for new reasons. Re-framing techniques (for example, as suggested above, re-framing 'giving in' as 'the way to win with ME') can provide them with a vital tool for coping with the negative attitudes which they are all-too-likely to encounter from others, but also the self-criticism which inability to overcome the symptoms of ME is likely to engender.

Once you have helped your client deal with the psychological adjustments needed to accept the fact that 'not fighting' is the best way to 'fight' this illness, you and/or your client may conclude that psychotherapy is not appropriate for them, and as a treatment for ME, it is not. However, your role may continue to be valuable as a witness and an audience for your client's developing strategies for survival and if possible, for long-term improvement. This may include assisting your client in considering any treatment they may care to try, either within or outside the normal medical settings, in as objective a way as possible.

Realistically, people who have ME need physical and practical help much more than they need psychotherapy, and they may rightly come to regard it as an optional extra.

Recommendations for the Medical Community

To enrich and expand effective treatment strategies, especially for chronic conditions, by beginning to include haemorheology within the medical canon and medical training.

It is a fundamental fact that every system in our body, every cell, requires oxygen and the removal of waste products in order to function. As a complete organism, without oxygen, we die. And each separate element of our body which lacks sufficient oxygen will become unable to carry out its intended function. The body's delivery system of oxygen to the cells consists of the red blood cells, which also remove waste products. Red blood cells need to be extremely deformable (flexible) in order to curl up and travel in the tiny capillaries which serve our muscles, brain and other organs. The physical properties of our red blood cells determine whether or not this function is carried out. It is very difficult, therefore, to understand why the subject of haemorheology (the physical properties of blood) is completely absent from medical training, medical textbooks, and medical journals. Dr. Simpson's numerous research papers, and his book, 'Blood Viscosity Factors – the Missing Dimension in Modern Medicine' [43] are ignored, to the detriment of any patient who has a condition which could be improved if blood viscosity issues were addressed. These conditions include diabetes, MS, ME, FM, Huntingdon's and Downs, among many others. This major omission from the general body of medical science needs to be rectified.

Naming

The major theme in Dr. Simpson's book is the need to identify ME, using Ramsay's original criteria, and give it a name which will clearly differentiate it from all the variations and labels which have been added since Ramsay's original work.

The New International Guidelines for the Diagnosis of ME, published in the Journal of Internal Medicine in July, 2011 set out clear criteria for diagnosis, and strongly recommend the creation of a completely separate category for ME, thereby effectively removing it from the much broader and heterogeneous category CFS (and from the treatment recommendations of the PACE Trial). It should be noted, however, that their criteria are not restricted to Ramsay's original ones. In Dr. Simpson's view this implies that all the conditions labelled CFS may wrongly be included.

Furthermore, as Dr. Simpson points out, remissions are a significant feature in Ramsay's definition and any proposed theory must account for them; yet remissions are not even mentioned in these, or other, guidelines.

Diagnostic protocols

Immediate diagnosis should be on the basis of the constellation of symptoms presented, their variability, and the exclusion of other possible conditions, including depression.

Medically, the fact that the symptoms, muscular, cognitive, and endocrine, are caused by changes in the shape population of red blood cells, depriving the tissues of oxygen and causing a build-up of waste products, should be recognised and addressed. (A micrograph of an *immediately-fixed* sample of blood can confirm that this is the situation.) Following confirmation of the diagnosis of ME, the steps recommended by Dr. Simpson for improving blood viscosity should be instigated.

A diagnosis of ME should be regarded as requiring an immediate and lengthy period of rest, ideally six months off work as a minimum, with the recommendation that all activities should be kept strictly limited.

ME treatment

A significant proportion of people who have ME will find their symptoms very much alleviated by one or another of the recommendations Dr. Simpson makes for addressing the problem of shape-changed red-blood cell populations. As mentioned elsewhere, these include Vitamin B12 as hydrocobalamin, pentoxifylline, 6g per day of fish oil, or 4 g per day of genuine EPO.

Complete inactivity will affect blood viscosity adversely, but virtually every official source of information about ME will state that exercise exacerbates symptoms. In the acute stage of this illness, even the most basic activities involved in self-care may already exceed what the patient is able to do without worsening of symptoms. Also, what can be undertaken one day may not be able to be performed on the next, and relapses caused by overexertion can be prolonged. This seems to be linked to the fact that the shift from aerobic to anaerobic muscle metabolism occurs very soon when a person with ME undertakes any form of exertion.

It continues to be the case that minimising physical exertion should be done sooner rather than later. In view of the fact that this is an illness which has the potential to lead to a long-term or permanent state of complete helplessness and dependency, diagnosis should be given quickly, and a diagnosis of ME should be treated as an extremely serious medical problem. **Rather than encouraging the patient to do as much as possible, the prescription must be the opposite, and this prescription should be given the weight that the possible prevention of serious disability requires.**

This is so completely contradictory to the views put forward by the group of psychiatrists who wield so much power in the field of ME, and apparently supported by the results of the PACE Trial, that we need to consider this document in more detail.

Response to the PACE trial

Apparently, the PACE Trial was undertaken to support the view that ME is a 'non-illness' which can be 'completely reversed' through changing the way people think, via Cognitive Behaviour Therapy, and forcing them to build up 'deconditioned' muscles through a program of exercise (Graded Exercise Therapy).

Interested parties include the NHS, the Department of Work and Pensions, and a range of insurance companies, many of whom employ the individuals who have either funded, designed, or carried out the study.

Obviously, as ME is an illness that is characterised by the relatively sudden appearance of multiple and severe disability, both muscular and cognitive, and it lasts a very long time, it is expensive to all of the above agencies if it is recognised as a physical illness (as it is by the World Health Organisation, which, as noted previously, categorises it as a neurological disorder).

A 'complete reversal' of this illness would save these organisations a lot of money. Actually, a complete reversal of this illness would be wonderful for the people who are suffering from it, a fact that seems to get lost among the controversy. Further, it would be reasonable to assume that patients for whom treatment had produced a 'complete reversal' would be a very vocal cohort in praise of whatever treatment had helped them. As far as I'm aware, no such cohort has yet been heard from.

The interests of the organisations which seek an effective treatment for ME because it is expensive to them, and the interests of people who have ME, are exactly the same. ME is expensive to people who get it, in terms of loss of jobs, loss of income, and the need for a great deal of personal assistance. It makes sense to stop pretending that it is psychological, and stop offering treatments which are very likely to make the illness more disabling and more long-lasting.

The plain fact of the matter is that, if the PACE Trial can be considered to have proved anything, it is that people who have ME are very physically ill people who spectacularly fail to respond to CBT and GET by getting back to anyone's definition of normal health.

Recommendations for Public Policy

Neither our thinking nor our legislation around disability is geared towards an illness that begins with severe disability, but can improve – ironically, improvement is proportional to how much the person has been able to behave like an invalid in the early stages! Most health policies and policies to do with disability presuppose either that a disability is permanent, or that an ill person may suffer from a progressively disabling illness which will end in their death.

A perfect example of this is the policy concerning acquiring a disability badge for car parking. In the early stages of ME, if the patient can get out in a car at all, on their own, they absolutely need to be parked close to where they need to be. A parking Blue Badge can make a real contribution towards improvement – the gradual lessening of disability. But the eligibility criteria for being allocated a Blue Badge sticker require that you are 'permanently' disabled. A constructive policy for a person with ME would be a disability parking sticker issued on a time-limited basis, to be reviewed periodically in the expectation that a point would be reached when it was no longer needed.

This approach could also be applied to the provision of disability living aids. For example, a physiotherapist and an occupational therapist should visit the patient's home with a view to teaching the client how to perform personal and household tasks with a minimum of physical exertion, and to re-organising his living arrangements so as to conserve physical and mental exertion. Aids and adaptations should be provided as for a very disabled person, but on a temporary basis, always with the assumption that these arrangements are intended to facilitate long-term recovery, when such modifications may no longer be needed and can be gradually withdrawn.

Contrary to the perverse labelling of people who have ME as suffering from 'somatoform symptom disorder', we are desperate to get back to our normal life – our professions, our educational activities, our role in our families. Given complete rest for the initial few months, followed by giving priority to every possible strategy and adaptation that can minimise physical exertion, we will do all we can to return to becoming contributing members of society as soon as we can. It seems perfectly apparent that the imposition of additional exertion in the name of 'treatment' could completely undermine these efforts and is the very opposite of what is required.

If insurers and governments want us to stop costing so much money, then they should give us what we need, right from the start. And stop spending money on centres and salaries based on the false belief that ME/CFS is a psychiatric problem, which offer ' treatments' that will prevent our recovery.

A SUMMARY OF SUGGESTIONS
FOR MANAGING YOUR OWN PROGRESS

What Dr. Simpson has to Say

Because it is possible for ME people to manage their disorder and to live relatively normal, albeit rather secluded lives, it is important to understand the main points of their health problem:

1. **ME is a problem of blood flow which differs from individual to individual, and may lead to dysfunction in a few or many parts of the body.**
2. **Lifestyles may be responsible for the exacerbation of symptoms.**
3. **Remission - brief or long term - may occur and blood flow patterns return to normal, but this does not mean that you are cured, and you remain at risk of relapse.**
4. **The primary problem involves obtaining a diagnosis of ME, as many physicians think in terms of CFS.**

The following suggestions have the objective of drawing attention to what ME sufferers can do for themselves.

As the usual daily activities will vary widely depending upon personal circumstances, such as living alone or having children to care for, this will determine your energy output. Therefore it is essential to intersperse periods of rest between parts of your activities of daily living. Endeavour to avoid long periods of bed rest, as this has an adverse effect on the flow properties of blood. In addition, with the objective of improving the physical properties of the blood, you should endeavour to fit in your daily programme a period of finite, low intensity activity. Daily walks to the nearest lamp post and back, at your own pace should continue for a week, then possibly doing the walk in both morning and afternoon. When you are comfortable with that level of activity, extend the walk to a second lamp post for a week at least, and thus extend your range.

Be aware of the adverse effects of both physical and mental stress. Both physical over exertion and emotional upsets and mental stress will have adverse effects on blood flow which would be additive to the ME-related changes in the blood and would trigger a relapse. So do not get involved in arguments and walk away from potentially stressful situations.

Both cigarette smoking and a diet rich in saturated fats lead to stiffening of red cells, so it is necessary to stop smoking and to adopt a low fat diet.

It has been found that in the early stages of acute ME, injections of 1ml of hydroxocobalamin at 10 to 14 day intervals were very helpful in 50% of cases, but it is not known why only 50% responded.

When the disorder progresses to chronic ME and hydroxocobalamin is no longer effective, there are three agents which could be helpful. However, it is not known which patients will respond to which treatment, but treatments should be taken for at least six weeks before deciding whether or not it was beneficial. If no benefits were identified try another agent.

The three agents are evening primrose oil (4 grams daily); fish oil (6 grams daily) pentoxifylline - a prescription drug (3 x 400 mg tabs daily).

Many ME people in different parts of the world have emailed to say how this programme has changed their lives.

What Nancy has to Say

Self-management begins with taking a firm grip on the fact that Ramsay's Disease (ME) requires that you just lie down for a while – quite a while – in the teeth of the fact that the entire culture around you insists that 'fighting' illness is the appropriate attitude to take, and that you should demonstrate this by making visible physical efforts to overcome the limitations of your illness. The cardinal feature of Ramsay's Disease (ME) – is that exertion, physical or mental, makes it worse. Pay attention! And insist that those around you pay attention, too. Trying to live a normal life, which is what you long to be able to do, requires rigid planning, ruthless attention to the conservation of your physical and mental resources for the activities which are most important to you. Take as much control as possible of your physical environment to this end, and take control as much as possible of the attitudes of those around you. Stay close to those who respect you and respect that you are doing your best. They need to understand that you will need a great deal of practical help to create the possibility of improvement, and of being able to continue to do at least some of your normal activities. Ask for it, accept it, and be gracious about it. You have always been the helper, you have a right to help right now, in order to have a chance to become the helper again in the future.

My basic advice can be put extremely briefly!

- The dietary supplements which Dr. Simpson recommends offer the best promise of significant improvement.

- If you are in the early stages, just keep lying down.
- You **must** conserve physical and mental energy right from the beginning if you want to have some hope of eventual improvement.

- It won't be easy to learn that 'giving in' is the only way to beat this illness, so you need to be a quick learner, and educate those around you, too.

- The way to 'fight' ME – Ramsay's Disease is to stop fighting!

Our very best wishes to you, as you navigate the complexities of Ramsay's Disease. We hope we have been helpful.

Nancy's references

[1] M. Ramsay, "Myalgic Encephalomyelitis: A Baffling Syndrome With a Tragic Aftermath," 1986. [Online]. Available: http://www.name-us.org/Definitions Pages/DefRamsay.htm. [Accessed 6 September 2012].

[2] A. M. Ramsay, Myalgic Encephalomyelitis and Postviral Fatigue States, the Saga of Royal Free disease, Second ed., The ME Association, 1988, Reprinted 2005, pp. 30-33.

[3] C. B. A. McEvedy, "Royal Free epidemic of 1955; a reconsideration," *British Medical Journal,* 3 January 1970.

[4] ME Association, "NHS specialist services throughout the UK," [Online]. Available: http://www.meassocition. or.uk/?page_id+1382. [Accessed 10 August 2012].

[5] R. C. Vermeulen, R. M. Kurk, F. C. Visser, W. Sluiter and H. R. Scholte, "Patients with chronic fatigue syndrome performed worse than controls in a controlled repeated exercise study despite a normal oxidative phosphorylation capacity.," *Journal of Translational Medicine,* vol. 8, no. 93, 2010.

[6] S. Finlay, "An illlness doctors don't recognise," *The Observer,* 1 June 1986.

[7] W. S. Harvey SB, "Chronic fatigue syndrome: identifying zebras amongst the horses," *BMC Medicine,* vol. 7, no. 58, 2009.

[8] G. K. J. A. C. T. S. M. White PD and P. T. M. Group, "Recovery from chronic fatigue syndrome after treatments given in the PACE trial," Cambridge University Press, 2013.

[9] M. E. W. M. Hooper M, "'Corporate Collusion? An overview of the misinformation about Myalgic Encephalomyelitis/Chronic Fatigue Syndrome arising from vested interests that pervades some UK Departments of State and other Agencies'," [Online]. Available: http://www.meactionuk.org.uk/Corporate_Collusion_2.htm. [Accessed 2012].

[10] G. SA, "How citation distortions create unfounded authority: Analysis of a citation network.," *British Medical Journal,* p. 339:b2680, 2009.

[11] P. M. Hooper, "Magical Medicine - Making an Illness Disappear," [Online]. Available: http://www.meactionuk.org.uk/magical-medicine.pdf. [Accessed 23 June 2012].

[12] C. K. G. S. W. S. T.-H. S. Jason LA, "Causes of Death Among Patients With Chronic Fatigue Syndrome," *Health Care for Women International,* vol. 27, no. 7, pp. 615-626, 2006.

[13] C. Wilson, "The Sophia Mirza Archive," [Online]. [Accessed 28 October 2012].

[14] ME Society of America, "Cardiac Insufficiency Hypothesis," [Online]. Available: http://www.cfids-cab.org/MESA. [Accessed 26 February 2013].

[15] M. T. F. Maes, "Why myalgic encephalomyelitis/chronic fatigue syndrome (ME/CFS) may kill you: disorders in the inflammatory and oxidative and nitrosative stress (IO&NS) pathways may explain cardiovascular disorders in ME/CFS," *Neuro Endocrinol Lett,* vol. 30, no. 6, pp. 677-693, 2009.

[16] F. M. M. Twisk, "A review on cognitive behavioral therapy (CBT) and graded exercise therapy (GET) in myalgic encephalomyelitis (ME)/chronic fatigue syndrome (CFS): CBT/GET is not only ineffective and not evidence-based, also potentially harmful for

many ME/CFS patients.," *Neuro Endocrinol Lett,* vol. 30, no. 3, pp. 284-299, 2009.

[17] A. L. M. Komaroff, "Review of The Psychopathology of Functional Somatic Syndromes by Peter Manu," *New England Journal of Medicine,* vol. 351, no. 26, pp. 2777-2778, 2003 December 2004.

[18] S. a. J. L. Song, "A population-based study of chronic fatigue syndrome (CFS) experienced in different patient groups: An effort to replicate Vercoulen et al's model of CFS," *Journal of Mental Health,* no. 14, pp. 277-289, 2005.

[19] T. F. Maes M, "Chronic fatigue syndrome: Harvey and Wessely's(bio)psychosocial model versus a bio(psychosocial) model based on inflammatory and oxidative and nitrosative stress pathways," 2010. [Online]. Available: http://www.biomedcentral.com/1741-7015/8/35.

[20] J. L. T.-H. S. Hawk C, "Differential diagnosis of chronic fatigue syndrome and major depressive disorder," *Int. J. Behav. Med.,* vol. 13, pp. 244-251, 2006.

[21] Hephaestus, *Articles on the Disgnostic and Statistical Manual of Mental Disorders, Including Diagnostic Inter view for DSM-IV, DSM-5.*

[22] "Allen Francis with Suzy Chapman - opposition to DSM5 SSD category," [Online]. Available: http://forums.phoenixrising.me.

[23] S. Chapman. [Online]. Available: http://www.dxrevisionwatch.com. [Accessed 1 March 2013].

[24] D. a. L. S. Pheby, "Risk factors for severe ME/CFS," *Biology and Medicine,* vol. 1, no. 4, pp. 50-74, 2009.

[25] D. A. J. Frances, "DSM5 In Distress - Mislabelling Medical Illness Mental Disorder," [Online]. Available: http://www.psychologytoday.com/blog/dsm5-in-distress/201212/mislabeling-medical-illness-mental-disorder. [Accessed 1 March 2012].

[26] A. (Beck, "Beck Depression Inventory," [Online]. Available: http://en.wikipedia.org/wiki/Beck_Depression_Inventory. [Accessed 21 August 2012].

[27] T. Courtney, "Queens refuse access to the PACE Trial raw data," 7 February 2013. [Online]. Available: http://www.meadvocacy.blogspot.co.uk. [Accessed 1 March 2013].

[28] M. M. Edlund, The Power of Rest - Why Sleep Alone Is Not Enough, New York: HarperOne, 2011.

[29] L. R. D. M. R. Paul, "Physiological cost of walking in those with chronic fatigue syndrome (CFS): A case-control study," *Disability and Rehabilitation,* vol. 31, no. 19, pp. 1593-1604, 2009.

[30] A. D. Acheson, "The clinical syndrome variously called benign myalgic encephalomyelitis, Iceland Disease and epidemic neuromyasthenia," in *The Clinical and Scientific Basis of Myalgic Encephalomyelitis/Chronic Fatigue Syndrome*, The Nightingale Foundation, 1992.

[31] K. H. S. M. P. J. B. G. Wiborg JF, "How does cognitive behaviour therapy reduce fatigue in patients with chronic fatigue syndrome: The role of physical activity'," *Psychological Medicine,* vol. 40, pp. 1281-87, 2010.

[32] M. Williams, "The Immunological Basis of ME/CFS: what is already known?," *The*

Journal of Invest in ME, vol. 6, no. 1, pp. 29-98, May 2012.

[33] U. C. f. D. C. (CDC), "Chronic Fatigue Syndrome," [Online]. Available: http://www.cdc/gov/cfs/general.

[34] P. M. Hooper, "Complaint to Editor of The Lancet about the PACE Trial Articles," March 2011. [Online]. Available: http://www.meactionuk.org.uk/COMPLAINT-to-Lancet-re-PACE.HTM. [Accessed 28 October 2012].

[35] S. Feehan, "Correspondence to Lancet re PACE," *Lancet,* pp. 1831-1832, 17 May 2011.

[36] A. Kewley, "Correspondence to Lancet re PACE," *Lancet,* pp. 1832-3, 17 May 2011.

[37] T. Kindlon, "Correspondence to Lancet re PACE," *Lancet,* vol. 377, p. 1833, 17 May 2011.

[38] B. v. d. S. M. Carruthers, "International Consensus Criteria for ME (Myalgic Encephalomyelitis)," *Journal of Internal Medicine,* 20 July 2011.

[39] P. S. Wessely, Interviewee, *Death Threats to ME Researchers.* [Interview]. 2 August 2011.

[40] R. J. S. B. W. Pech, "Organisational sociopaths: rarely challenged, often promoted. Why?," *Society and Business Review,* vol. 2, no. 3, pp. 254-269, 2007.

[41] M. P. Stout, "Inside the Mind of a Sociopath," in *The Sociopath Next Door: The Ruthless vx. the Rest of Us*, New York, Broadway Books, 2005.

[42] D. D. Rutherford, "Chronic fatigue syndrome (Myalgic encephalimyelitis)," [Online].

[43] D. L. O. Simpson, Blood Viscosity Factors - The Missing Dimension to Modern Medicine, Highlands, New Jersey: Mumford Institute, pp. 247-263.